THE CULT OF CROSSFIT

The Cult of CrossFit

*Christianity and the
American Exercise Phenomenon*

Katie Rose Hejtmanek

NEW YORK UNIVERSITY PRESS
New York

NEW YORK UNIVERSITY PRESS
New York
www.nyupress.org

© 2025 by New York University
All rights reserved

Please contact the Library of Congress for Cataloging-in-Publication data.

ISBN: 9781479831784 (hardback)
ISBN: 9781479831814 (paperback)
ISBN: 9781479831838 (library ebook)
ISBN: 9781479831821 (consumer ebook)

This book is printed on acid-free paper, and its binding materials are chosen for strength and durability. We strive to use environmentally responsible suppliers and materials to the greatest extent possible in publishing our books.

Manufactured in the United States of America

10 9 8 7 6 5 4 3 2 1

Also available as an ebook

For those living in the wake and trying to imagine an otherwise

CONTENTS

Introduction: CrossFit as Americana 1

1. A Cult, a Community, a Religion Run by a Biker Gang 21

2. Salvation through Bearing One's Daily Cross(Fit) 39

3. CrossFit Capitalism: Oracles and Garages 59

4. CrossFit and the American Frontier Spirit 81

5. Heroes and Sheroes 103

6. Science, CrossFit Style 125

7. This Was Not the Apocalypse We Trained For! 150

Conclusion 171

Acknowledgments 179

Glossary 183

Notes 185

Bibliography 199

Index 217

About the Author 227

Introduction

CrossFit as Americana

In a 2015 *60 Minutes* segment titled "King of CrossFit," correspondent Sharyn Alfonsi begins the main portion narrating, "Last summer the finals of the CrossFit Games were broadcast on ESPN. Forty-five thousand people showed up to watch the contestants, who look like superheroes, heave, jump, and lift until a champion was crowned."[1] "Rich Froning is the fittest man in history!" is heard from the ESPN broadcast that is playing as Alfonsi narrates. Alfonsi continues, "If this is the body that defines a new kind of fitness, the brain that dreamt it all up belongs to Greg Glassman. Well before CrossFit was a competition, he designed it as a new way to workout. He says it can transform anyone, and he's not just talking about bulging biceps and six-pack abs."

"I'll deliver you to your genetic potential," Glassman states, with his sunglasses perched on top of a baseball cap turned backward. Alfonsi is now interviewing Glassman in a CrossFit gym.

"Your genetic potential?" Alfonsi asks incredulously.

"Yeah," he continues.

"Sounds like you're creating a robot or something," Alfonsi remarks.

Pointing to a white woman in black leggings and a pale-blue tank top, with her blond hair in a messy bun, who is cleaning (or lifting a barbell up to her shoulders) and push-jerking a few reps, Glassman declares, "Look at her. She was meant to look like that. That's what nature would have carved from her a million years ago. Or she'd have been eaten." He emphasizes certain words for effect, chuckling at the end.

Alfonsi continues, narrating, "Glassman hardly looks like an exercise guru. There's no hint of ripped muscle underneath his untucked shirt. But he's widely considered the most powerful man in fitness today. Glassman is the architect of CrossFit, a workout program that mixes elements of weightlifting, calisthenics, and gymnastics. The classes take place in what CrossFitters call a 'box,' a stripped-down, willfully ugly space. The exercises range from simple to sadistic and made Greg Glassman, a college dropout, a multimillionaire."

Back in interview format, Alfonsi states, "You didn't invent weightlifting. You didn't invent calisthenics. You didn't invent gymnastics."

Glassman replies with a blasé "Nope" to each assertion.

Alfonsi asks in earnest, "So what did you do?"

"I invented that doing lateral raises and curls while eating pretzels is dumb. That's what I invented."

According to Glassman, gym owners have long ignored the importance of diet, all too happy to watch their members fall into a trance on the treadmill.

The narration continues, "CrossFit classes usually don't take more than an hour. Athletes compete against each other and the clock. To keep their energy up, they're encouraged to follow something called a paleo diet, heavy on meats and vegetables—food fit for a caveman."

"I've heard you say CrossFit prepares you for the 'unknown and unforeseen.' It sounds like you're getting ready to go to war," Alfonsi states.

Glassman responds, "Yeah, why not? For getting ready for war, getting ready for earthquake [sic], getting ready for mugging [sic], getting ready for the horrible news that you have leukemia. What awaits us all is challenge. That's for sure."

* * *

CrossFit in the United States has become an increasingly popular fitness regimen and sport, one predicated on a survivalist, militaristic approach. US fitness has often been linked with the US military, but CrossFit has imbued military and life-or-death meaning into its training regimen. It claims to train participants as if they were Navy SEALs preparing for disaster, war, or the apocalypse, and it names its workouts after US soldiers who have died during the war on terror. But CrossFit also claims to be many other things—a business, a brand, a fitness regimen, a community, a sport that crowns the fittest man and woman on Earth, a cult, the best hour of one's day—and to offer its members salvation. American CrossFit, infused with these meanings, has developed a fascinating culture centered on the workout's tremendous difficulty, the program's cult-like nature, and its organization of everyday life for the people who are devoted to it.

CrossFit appeals to people from various walks of American life. I know a CrossFit gym that operates a transgender powerlifting club where people use CrossFit and heavy lifting as a method of healing from sexual violence and trauma.[2] At the same time, Marjorie Taylor Greene is an avid CrossFitter who owned a CrossFit gym before becoming a Far Right Trump-supporting congresswoman. There are self-identified Christian CrossFit gyms. There are Black-owned CrossFit gyms. There are women-owned and veteran-owned CrossFit gyms. There are Cross-Fit gyms filled with elite CrossFitters who compete at the CrossFit Games, the annual international competition organized by CrossFit headquarters (HQ), which the winner is crowned as "Fittest on Earth." There are CrossFit gyms in high schools and CrossFit gyms geared toward senior citizens. And that is just in the United States. There are also CrossFit gyms in 162 countries and on seven continents; CrossFit Deep Freeze is located at McMurdo Station, a US research station, in Antarctica (although its last Facebook post was from 2016).

One of the fastest growing businesses of all time, CrossFit has found success in the United States (and beyond) by being what the sociologist Marcelle Dawson calls a "reinventive institution," or something that encourages voluntary commitment to self-reinvention or self-improvement.[3] By encouraging voluntary self-improvement, CrossFit as a leisure brand taps into American values of hard work and moral goodness.[4]

In the United States, "religion" is often colloquially used as a framework to make sense of commitment to a set of beliefs and practices linking moral goodness with hard work.[5] "Religion" is endlessly used to talk about CrossFit. Everyone knows this is a metaphor, an exaggeration, and yet it is also a sincere framework that journalists, scholars, and CrossFitters use to make sense of the way people are drawn to and engage in the sport and fitness regime of CrossFit.[6] What makes Americans so casually use "religion" to make sense of something like CrossFit? Perhaps it is because the religious resonances of American CrossFit are not simply panreligious. These American values come from Christian values and norms that permeate life in the United States.[7] It is because of the United States' Christian roots and legacies that such seemingly offhanded remarks about CrossFit—such as, "it's a cult!"—make sense.

Finding elements of Christianity in a supposedly secular practice of fitness illustrates how forms of Christianity become subtle: saying "bless you" after sneezes, using Jesus Christ's birthday to determine the year (for both AD and CE), watching redemption stories in Hollywood movies, or the ubiquity of the apocalypse in American social life. These subtle forms of Christianity are like what the American studies and Black studies scholar Christina Sharpe calls "the weather" or a total environment, something pervasively in the air.[8] They also make up what the anthropologist James Wertsch calls the underlying codes that shape American national identity.[9] I call these subtle forms of Christianity, these underlying "religious" codes that make up "the weather" in American social life, *cultural Christianity*.

Cultural Christianity

Cultural Christianity, or the expansive and often obscured legacies of Christianity in contemporary American life, can be traced and understood using theories of history and cultural knowledge.

Sharpe proposes a framework called "the wake," which includes the track left by a ship on the water's surface, a ritual of death, or raised consciousness.[10] The wake left by a ship through water is useful for us here. This wake symbolizes elements of the past that are not really past; they still linger, rupturing the present as ripple effects long after the ship has sailed into the horizon.[11] Sharpe writes that *thinking* about life in the US needs to stay in the wake as a way to make sense of "encountering a past that is not past," to understand how the past continues to rupture and ripple through the present.[12] Thinking about CrossFit needs to stay in the wake of Christianity to fully understand it and how people make sense of it.

This thinking relies on the English poet and critical studies scholar Dionne Brand's explanation of history: "One enters a room and history follows; one enters a room and history precedes. History is already seated in the chair in the empty room when one arrives. Where one stands in a society seems always related to this historical experience." She calls this "sitting in the room with history."[13] One of the histories that sits with us in this book is American Christianity—American Christianity as it was forged in the early settling of the North American continent by people seeking a New Jerusalem, American Christianity as it has transformed through a variety of awakenings, movements, splinters, schisms, and theologies that emerged in the social, political, and economic contexts throughout the founding, solidifying, and changing American national experiment. This book illustrates how "religion" and Christianity sit already in the CrossFit gym.

However, this history does not look the same over time. American Christianity is different today than it was in the 1600s, 1770s, 1840s, or 1950s. Therefore, I use the cultural historian and African American studies scholar Saidiya Hartman's understanding of an "afterlife" to make sense of Christianity's morphing staying power. Hartman writes that slavery "established a measure and a ranking of life and worth that has yet to be undone," leaving its afterlives in the skewed life chances of people living in the Americas.[14] I use this understanding of "afterlives" to *think* about the way Christianity, entrenched centuries ago, has yet to be undone, leaving formally religious and seemingly secular afterlives in the US.[15] We will explore how Christianity's afterlives are at work in CrossFit in the United States. These afterlives include calling CrossFit a "religion" and the various ways cultural Christianity appears in the stories, communities, capitalisms, science, and preparations for the future that occur in American CrossFit gyms.[16]

Therefore, this book is as much an interrogation of American culture as it is an examination of CrossFit. Indeed, CrossFit's success offers a window into the way American historical afterlives find purchase in the twenty-first century—often through stories.

CrossFit Stories

CrossFit tells many stories about itself, including the one on *60 Minutes* mentioned at the beginning of the chapter. Part of the episode detailed its origins story. Alfonsi relates that after dropping out of college, Glassman "became a personal trainer and started experimenting with some of the exercises that would become the backbone of his creation. His workouts were loud and disruptive, and gym owners were not impressed."

"How many gyms did you get tossed out of?" Alfonsi asks during their interview.

"About five or six or seven," Glassman responds.

"You don't like being told what to do," Alfonsi replies.

"Oh, I don't mind being told what to do. I just won't do it," Glassman chuckles. "Say anything you want."

The narration continues, "He opened his own gym in Santa Cruz in 2001. Today there are twelve thousand CrossFit boxes around the world, each one defiantly barren. The company is private but estimated to be worth hundreds of millions of dollars, and Greg Glassman owns 100 percent of it. He has no board of directors and says he never had a business plan. But he recently found himself at Harvard Business School, where he was invited to share the secrets of CrossFit's meteoric growth."

In a video of Glassman at Harvard, he attests, "If you like metrics, you like money. We are the fastest growing large chain on Earth. We have broken all records."

"I'm not trying to grow a business. I'm doing the right things for the right people for the right reasons," Glassman tells Harvard.

"One reason CrossFit's grown so fast is because just about anyone who wants to open a box can, after paying a $3,000 yearly fee and passing a two-day seminar. It's how the company makes most of its money," Alfonsi narrates.

"Two days to take a course, then I can open a gym?" Alfonsi follows up in the interview.

"Amazing, huh?" Glassman replies.

"I mean, to me, is that enough?" she asks.

"Well, here's the alternative. Here's what it used to be. All you had to have was the money, and you don't even have to take a test. That's where every other chain came from. Someone just launched them."

"And unlike most gym chains," Alfonsi narrates, "Glassman—a die-hard libertarian—relinquishes nearly all control over his affiliates. They can open a box next door to another box if they want. It's probably not surprising Glassman believes the strongest one will survive."

* * *

In these first few minutes of "King of CrossFit," Glassman and Alfonsi hit on several key notes in the story of CrossFit: a die-hard libertarian, college-dropout personal trainer kicked out of regular gyms for his rogue style of training created a new workout regimen designed to deliver one's genetic potential. This regimen is used to build superhero-like bodies prepared for disaster and forged through functional fitness, performed in a defiantly barren gym, while eating like a caveman.

Local CrossFit gyms also tell CrossFit stories on their web and Facebook pages. CrossFitters share many stories with one another and with non-CrossFitters. One of the oldest jokes about CrossFit is, "The first rule of CrossFit: talk about CrossFit." This joke references and inverts the critically acclaimed movie *Fight Club*'s first rule (don't talk about fight club) at the same time that it demands that stories about CrossFit be told. This book examines the stories told by CrossFit and CrossFitters, exploring how they build on common American themes to give weight and credence to the fitness practice. In the *60 Minutes* episode, we hear a few of these American themes: through hard work, one can realize one's dreams, such as being an entrepreneur and owning a CrossFit gym or having a body that both looks good and is strong and capable, even hero-like. CrossFit taps into common American myths such as that the American Dream can be realized through bootstrap/hard-work capitalism and a belief in one's exceptional abilities. These are what Wertsch calls "national narrative projects" (NNPs): the storytelling we do that reinforces the ideas we have about who we are as a national society. These NNPs help us to create communities, understand ourselves, and make sense of the lives we live.[17] They are the *official stories* that Americans tell about ourselves, that we all know, and that feel right when we live them out.

However, Wertsch argues that in addition to overt narrative projects, there are also underlying codes—what he calls "narrative templates"— that shape what stories make sense and feel right. These underlying codes frame who we are and what we think, feel, and believe, but their origins are elusive; they are covert, in contrast to the overt NNPs. These underlying codes are removed from conscious daily life and emerge in the wake or afterlives of the official stories that are deeply embedded in our minds and bodies.

For example, in the *60 Minutes* interview and imagery, all the "superheroes" at the CrossFit Games or in the local CrossFit gym where the video for the episode takes place are white, young, able-bodied, and conventionally attractive. They can afford to commit to a protein-rich diet and workout regimen that "delivers to them their genetic potential."

The underlying code here is the implicit link among fitness, white bodies, and exceptionalism. This link between superheroes, whiteness, and genetic potential can come off in other contexts as a narrative project for ethnonationalists, white supremacists, and racists. In the *60 Minutes* video, neither Glassman nor Alfonsi makes this connection. But it is still there, subtly in the background video, operating as a covert story, an underlying code, an afterlife of whom the American Dream was meant to serve. In fact, most Americans would not readily claim to hold white supremacist values as their own. They might even claim the opposite is true as an official American story or NNP: we are a country of immigrants where anyone can tap into their rugged individualism to realize the American Dream or their genetic potential. But the CrossFit story that taps into these desires and dreams comes from historical legacies, bringing with it underlying codes that work on us covertly and unconsciously. These underlying codes operate in the background, in the wake of hundreds of years of linking exceptionalism with God's chosen people, the white, male, Christian American meant to win the West (and other imperialistic battles) through heroic individualism, vigilante justice, and Manifest Destiny.

This book examines both kinds of stories—official national narrative projects and narrative templates—to reveal the overt and covert ways in which CrossFit reflects the afterlives of settler Christian colonialism apparent in the contemporary US.

But CrossFit is not just about the stories it tells; it is also about the way people move. In fact, the stories become meaningful through the workouts themselves, in the daily commitment to "the CrossFit methodology." You can't understand CrossFit just by its stories; you must do it as well. Therefore, to write this book about CrossFit, I had to put my body on the line.

Doing and Researching CrossFit, Anthropology Style

In 2016, I began pilot research on CrossFit, Strongman, weightlifting (one word means the sport, two words mean general strength training), and powerlifting. I was interested in new things I was seeing: shirts that read, "Strong Is the New Sexy" and "Strong Is the New Skinny," and muscular female mannequins at the sporting goods stores. As someone built for strength and power with more muscles than a woman "should" have (unless she is an elite gymnast or sprinter), I was interested in this new shift. I am relatively "straight sized," meaning normal-size women's clothing fits me, but my thighs have always been a bit too big and my back a bit too broad for any single size of mass-produced clothing. I had been a gymnast and a sprinter, though despite state championships and records in high school, I would not call myself elite. My athletic career was cut short by two back surgeries by the time I was nineteen; the second one fused my last vertebra with my sacrum. While I spent most of my twenties rehabbing from that serious surgery, I never lost the girth in my quads, the strength in my legs, or the ability to do a handful of pull-ups in a row. As someone who felt she had had her athletic career stolen from her, I jumped at the chance to investigate the rise of the new strength sports.

I reached out to a few CrossFit gym owners in New York City to ask if they would be interested in having an anthropologist hang around. I am a professor at Brooklyn College of the City University of New York and wanted to focus my research on gyms close to home. One gym owner—I'll call him Paul—asked me to come in for his gym's free class for the CrossFit curious.[18] I had been racing track and field for a few years prior to this research, including on elite relay teams. In fact, one of my relay-mates went to the 2016 Rio Olympics in the Heptathlon. I was the slowest on this fast team: a mid-to-late-thirties white college professor who was making up for lost time. But I had been on the track practicing my sport and in the gym strength training to be faster. So, when the CrossFit gym owner asked me to come through for the freebie workout, I was game. I appreciated a workout as part of an interview to assess my abilities and commitment.

The CrossFit-curious workout was an hour long; we were taught a few new skills and then put through a MetCon. (There will be a whole slew of CrossFit words to know in this book. I have made a list in appendix A). "MetCon" is short for "metabolic conditioning," the timed CrossFit "workout of the day," or "WOD." The MetCon that Paul put us through was "for time" (i.e., as fast as you can) three rounds of five pull-ups and a 270-meter run. The 270 meters was up the block to the street and back through the rolled-up garage door. We were instructed to "scale" or modify pull-ups to make fifteen doable. Coach Paul suggested that I use a short box and jump to do the pull-ups. All five of us in the class were told which pull-up bar we would use, and we organized our stations to fit our scaling needs. Coach Paul asked if we were ready; I nodded as I stood on my twenty-inch box, prepared for the "on your marks, get set, go" of the starting blocks. Instead, he started the CrossFit gym clock, which counts down from ten, with the three, two, and one, accompanied by a beep and then a longer beep on the "Go!" CrossFit has trademarked this "3 . . . 2 . . . 1 . . . Go!" With the longer beep, I jumped up five times very quickly, feeling a bit like I was cheating, and then jumped off the box and raced out the garage door, up the block, and back again; I finished all three rounds in no time. This WOD was in my wheelhouse, as they say. Not only did my sprint training include 300-meter repeats, but my gym workout regularly included multiple sets of ten strict pull-ups. If this was a test to see if I could study CrossFit, I had passed. I would later learn that Coach Paul informed his coaches that they would have an anthropologist hanging around and that "she's really fit."[19]

But as any CrossFitter knows, it is the things that are not in your wheelhouse that need your attention. I had to learn to squat below parallel, to deadlift with proper form, to perform the Olympic lifts (the snatch and the clean and jerk), to kip and butterfly (use momentum) my pull-ups, to string double-unders (the CrossFit method of jumping rope) together, and so many other tasks. I am built and had been training for speed; my very first Fran time (one of the named workouts called "The Girls," which consists of thrusters, a barbell skill where the barbell is caught in a deep squat and then thrust overhead, and pull-ups in sequence) was four minutes and twenty-four seconds doing mostly strict pull-ups. But anything over five minutes and I got overheated and red-faced and wondered why I had chosen to do this research and if it was too late to change it. But I didn't change my project. I changed my body. My body went from specializing in sprinting to being generally fit, the CrossFit way. I did this by spending extensive time at two CrossFit gyms in Brooklyn and one in Manhattan for over two years. In 2017, I attended and passed a Level 1 Training Course, a CrossFit course required for all CrossFit coaches and CrossFit gym owners. I conducted this research from April 2016 to June 2018, finishing the bulk of my participant observation in the United States at a CrossFit gym's all-women powerlifting meet.

In addition to the deep ethnographic research on CrossFit in New York City, I also visited CrossFit gyms throughout the United States and around the world. I have family in Alabama, Chicago, Seattle, and New Mexico and regularly visited CrossFit gyms when there for holidays and semester breaks. In August 2018, I went to Delhi, India, for ten weeks to study CrossFit there. I then traveled to Melbourne, Australia, in November for another ten weeks of CrossFit research. I passed through Hong Kong on the way and did a few days of research there. During my various travels from 2016 to the present day, I have "dropped in," the CrossFit phrase for stopping at a local CrossFit gym while away from home, at gyms in Paris, France; Cusco, Peru; two in Marrakesh, Morocco; and anywhere I could find a local CrossFit gym. I visited mainstream gyms in all these places as well, comparing CrossFit gyms with other local fitness practices. I have been to a CrossFit gym on six continents. CrossFit Deep Freeze is on my bucket list. Once I returned from my international research, I spent a few more months examining CrossFit in the United States. I paid particular attention to what, after cross-cultural research, seemed *very American*.

To make sense of this doing CrossFit workouts, I rely on several French theorists—Pierre Bourdieu, Michel Foucault, and Marcel Mauss—who argue that it is through subjecting the body to daily habits, techniques, or practices that we give meaning to the stories we tell.[20] Culture gets into us as we "practice" being a person in a cultural milieu. Cultural norms, values, ideas, and histories can thus be found in our bodies, in our behaviors, feelings, and feelings about our behaviors. The anthropologist Thomas Csordas calls this "embodiment," which is based on "somatic modes of attention."[21] Somatic modes of attention are the ways we attend to the world in our bodies, which enables our bodies to be the existential ground of culture; culture is not "out there" in the world but lived out, in, and through our bodies.[22] The anthropologist Brenda Farnell argues that this somatic attention requires that we understand not just that the body feels things or gives attention to things but how the body moves.[23] Her book's subtitle is "I Move Therefore I Am," a play on Descartes's "I think therefore I am." Body movement is communicative: the body "talks" through movement. *Doing* CrossFit is communicating many things—to the person doing the CrossFitting, to others who also do it, to the public trying to make sense of this way of doing exercise. I argue that much of what is communicated are deeply felt and believed American values, stories, and ideologies.

I spent years studying CrossFit using my body as a methodological tool.[24] I transformed my body and mind through CrossFit: I gained new muscle, lost some fat, and developed "mental fitness" by learning to manage anxiety and fear in the workouts. I stopped sprinting and focused on learning the skills and training logic of CrossFit. It is because of my experience in other sports and with other fitness practices that I can see some of the subtle differences between CrossFit, general fitness routines, and other kinds of painful sport training. CrossFit is about the "practice" of it.

I use this framework of practice as both theory and method. CrossFit is a fitness regimen that requires consistent body work such as attending class, building strength, and doing a WOD. But then there are deep cultural meanings ascribed to this daily exercise regimen. For example, a painful workout with forms of movement (such as squats and other "functional movements") builds a CrossFit body, and these workouts shape the mind and heart so that these painful workouts are understood as good for us, meaningful, and part of the important, unique work of what it means to be a CrossFitter. Attending to the pain in my body during a workout but then pushing through that pain with a group of others doing the same creates a community of fellow sufferers who find deep meaning in this practice. This book is about these deep cultural meanings. And they can't be understood without the doing. Therefore, not only did I have to study what people were doing, but I had to do it myself.

I also observed other people doing CrossFit. I would hang out at the gym all day long, watching waves of people come in for morning, noon, and evening classes. I watched CrossFit classes for people over fifty-five years old and the CrossFit class for new moms and babies, where a babysitter watched the babies while the moms did the WOD. I watched "Friday Night Lights," a local weekly competition that happened during the Fridays of the CrossFit Open, the first round of the CrossFit Games that is held at local gyms worldwide and where CrossFitters competed for fitness glory at their respective gyms. I did intensive observation for over two years in the US and then for months in India and Australia. We cultural anthropologists call our method "participant observation," where we aim to get both an inside and outside observer's perspective. I would attend parties and potlucks, go get beers or coffee with people after class, hang out at the park, go to local competitions across town, and so on.

I also asked people to fill out a questionnaire and sit down for interviews. I interviewed coaches, gym owners, former coaches, recently converted CrossFitters, gym "OGs," as they are called (or long-term members), people who were the best in the gym, and those who did CrossFit in their final days despite debilitating illness. I interviewed men and women, corporate lawyers and elementary school teachers, Wall Street traders and philosophy professors, theater folk and college athletes, Marines and Innocence Project lawyers, New Yorkers and folks from Wyoming. CrossFitters come from all walks of life, and I was able to ask what CrossFit means to a wide range of people.

While I currently live in New York City, I was born in Colorado and raised in Wyoming. I grew up riding horses, hiking, and fishing in the mountains on the weekends. Our fresh or pickled vegetables came from our backyard garden, and our meat, from something my father hunted and killed (and hung in the garage before taking it to the local butcher). I went to Girl Scout camp and earned ribbons at the county and state fairs in 4-H sewing and cooking. In college, I majored in anthropology but also took courses in the College of Agriculture, excelling in my Rangeland Management class despite being the only one not wearing Wranglers or cowboy boots. After college, I worked under the anthropologist Marc Boglioli, who studied hunting in Vermont, for the University of Wyoming (my alma mater) on a United States National Forest Service grant.[25] We researched and documented the various historical uses of publicly held lands. This included learning the different histories of the Colorado and Wyoming frontier as told by Eastern Shoshone and Northern Arapahoe elders, German pioneers, Basque and Mexican sheep farmers, Mormon settlers, Chinese immigrants, Texas cattle ranchers, outlaws, US presidents, and other people who made their way across the Rocky Mountains.[26] I then moved to St. Louis, Missouri, and paid attention to the frontier history of the "Gateway to the West." Thus, my understanding of America's wake, stories, underlying codes, and afterlives does not just come from New York City or the academy but also from horseback in the least populated state in the country.[27]

Although CrossFitters come from all walks of life, they do skew one way. According to Rally Fitness, based on demographic data on the

CrossFit website, CrossFitters are generally elite, white members of US society.[28] Forty percent of CrossFitters have postgraduate degrees. Eighty-six percent of CrossFitters are white, and over half have an annual income greater than $150,000. Sixty-one percent are between the ages of twenty-five and forty-five, and they are split down the middle with regard to gender. The cost of a CrossFit gym membership is notoriously high, creating a cost-of-entry barrier for many who might wish to join but cannot afford it. CrossFit is considered a "boutique" fitness brand because of this. A simple Google search of "Why is CrossFit so expensive?" will reveal pages of articles written on the topic; it is common knowledge that CrossFit is expensive.[29] My average monthly CrossFit membership (across three gyms in New York City) was $275 a month, with a teacher discount. At the same time, I paid $125 a month for a Chelsea Piers Sports Club membership (a premier sports facility), also with a teacher discount. CrossFit gym-goers are also members of the armed forces or military without college degrees; some receive gym-supplied scholarships due to economic need, and some are people of color with money to spend. However, the demographics are clear: American CrossFitters are, by and large, highly educated, well paid, and white. I also fit most of these demographics, as I am a white college professor with a PhD.

This demographic can be seen in a lot of the media produced by CrossFit, which I also used as data for this book.[30] CrossFit has produced a lot of media: documentaries, journals, the Games, and too many to count short videos found on the CrossFit website. Greg Glassman, the cofounder of CrossFit, has done many formal interviews, including at Harvard Divinity School, Harvard Business School, the National War College, and the annual State Policy Network Conference. I use these interviews, journal articles, feature-length films, and short instructive videos as data as well. Many articles have been written about CrossFit, and I draw on ones from the *New York Times*, *Time, Inc.*, *New York*, *Men's Health*, *Christianity Today*, and other news sources as data for this book. CrossFitters have written books, blog posts, testimonials, and workout strategies, and I tap into all of it as data as well.[31]

I also compare what CrossFitters in India, Peru, Morocco, and Australia said about CrossFit and fitness, why they do CrossFit, and what they think translates well from the original American version to cross-cultural contexts. CrossFit is a worldwide phenomenon, with over six thousand gyms outside the US. But it became clear through my cross-cultural research and collaborations with non-American scholars studying and writing about CrossFit that its culturally Christian elements do not travel well. They are an American phenomenon.

In the US, exercising at a gym can come to be and feel like Christianity, despite people's best efforts *not* to be religious or Christian. Throughout the book, I illustrate how many afterlives of Christianity emerge as meaningful in American CrossFit gyms, stories, and experiences. CrossFit is a window into how Christian histories are already in the rooms/gyms/stories with us, as a past that is not past, the wake that remains, or an underlying code that Americans embody.

I wrapped up my CrossFit participant observation with Murph—a mile run, three hundred squats, two hundred push-ups, one hundred pull-ups, and a mile run—on May 31, 2019, completing the Hero WOD in thirty-eight minutes and twenty-five seconds, in a fourteen-pound vest and judged by another CrossFit coach, Coach Peter. When I began, I could barely do anything over four minutes, and I finished my research with a Murph time in the ninetieth percentile, something I never thought possible in 2016.[32] I completed this workout and then switched to training and competing in Olympic weightlifting (and became a world and national champion in my weight class and age group). I continue to "drop in" at CrossFit gyms but only to train for weightlifting, not to take a class. In other words, I didn't commit to CrossFit. I am not a die-hard CrossFitter. I like it, I can do it, I spent years of my life trying to understand it, and my aim is to represent it accurately, but I wasn't "saved" by CrossFit. We will see how the idea of salvation through CrossFit, with its militaristic approach and violent intensity, is a particularly American rendition of a Christian plotline.

Serious Popular Culture

The professor of comparative religion David Chidester argues in his book *Authentic Fakes* that popular culture is often seen as "play" and not "serious" as a topic of academic research.[33] The anthropologists Niko Besnier, Susan Brownell, and Thomas Carter write in their book on sport that sport is "easy to dismiss as an inconsequential aspect of our lives."³⁴ The professor of history Natalia Petrzela wrote a piece for the *Chronicle of Higher Education* discussing how she felt compelled to keep her gym life separate from her scholarship (she has since written a book-length history of exercise in the US) because "wellness is a dirty word" in the academy.³⁵ For many people, academic interest in the physical emerges when something goes wrong, such as chronic pain or changes in physical abilities.³⁶ Sport, popular culture, and exercise are seen as unserious aspects of people's lives, definitely less serious than religion, education, politics, history, or literature. But they are meaningful. Many Americans think about and participate in sport or fitness. They are avenues where power operates and people make meaning in their lives.³⁷

This book illustrates how CrossFit is a window into how America's histories and wakes are lived out, even at the gym. Like Besnier, Brownell, and Carter's claim about sport, I find that exercise can be easily dismissed as either a "fact" of biological human need or an inconsequential aspect of our lives. But it isn't. In fact, I argue, it is a primary way that American values, ideologies, hierarchies, and histories get built into our bodies, one workout at a time.

Take the American superhero. Academic scholarship examines how American myths and fantasies, built on Christian frameworks, make their way into superhero movies, video games, and comic books. This book shows how CrossFit moves the superhero frameworks out of the realm of fantasy—such as reading comics or watching movies—and into the bodies of CrossFitters, through everyday exercise and explicitly named CrossFit Hero Workouts.

Akin to Chidester and those who study the American superhero, I examine the way "religion" as a framework gets mapped onto popular culture. In the United States, this religion is Christianity, specifically white Protestant Christianity. I am not the first to make the claim that Christian frameworks undergird American social life. Famous scholars have claimed that the American work ethic and US capitalism are founded on the Protestant ethic (Max Weber) and that US democracy is predicated on US Christianity (Alexis de Tocqueville).³⁸ In fact, Tocqueville argued that "there is no country in the whole world in which the Christian religion retains a greater influence over the souls of men than in America."³⁹ These scholars wrote about the US in the late nineteenth and early twentieth centuries. The United States has undergone radical transformations since the nineteenth century, when Weber and Tocqueville were writing about the US as a Christian nation. Therefore, the shape of Christianity's wake has changed, but the existence of the wake has not.

The leading sociologist of religion Christian Smith argues that the institutions—economic, political, legal, and educational—that undergird American life have been modernized and secularized since the 1870s.[40] Pew Research illustrates that a significantly higher percentage of the population no longer identifies as Christian, becoming "Nones" (those who do not officially identify with a religious tradition).[41] These data have led many people to believe that the US is becoming less Christian and understood as a secular modern nation-state.[42]

However, I found that cultural Christianity still shapes supposedly secular popular culture practices like CrossFit. Therefore, even if people don't *identify* as Christian as much anymore, the wake of culturally Christian values and ideologies influences much of everyday life. The educator and social activist Paul Kivel calls this "Christian hegemony," which refers to "the everyday, systemic set of Christian values, individuals and institutions that dominate all aspects of US society," and it continues to organize American life in overt (NNP) and covert (narrative template) ways.[43] For example, post-9/11 wars were framed as crusades (a specific Christian reference to medieval wars against Muslims in the Middle East), and the US has been referred to by politicians from John F. Kennedy to Mitt Romney to Joe Biden as a "city upon a hill," a reference to a 1630 sermon by the Puritan John Winthrop in Massachusetts, preaching from the Gospel of Matthew.[44] Cultural Christianity is the history that sits with us, already there.

As the national surveys suggest, fewer people identify as Christian. But Christianity has not gone away; it has become less an identity we select, less religious tradition, and more the wake, afterlives, the history already in the room. Cultural Christianity continues to hold great influence over Americans, perhaps less in the churches and more in the gyms.

CrossFit as a voluntary commitment to self-improvement is understood to be virtuous. The philosopher Alasdair MacIntyre writes in his text on virtue, "The only criteria for success or failure in a human life as a whole are the criteria of success or failure in a narrated or to-be-narrated quest," and that quest is for a good life.[45] Virtue is not universal. What makes a "good life" or the "narrative quest" that describe it are not universal. They are cultural. To live a virtuous life is to live in accordance with narratives or stories about what a good person should be. It is making sense of one's life within the larger narrative frameworks that one has been born into, has grown into, and *feels* are the *right* ways to live. CrossFit provides an example of how the narrative quest for the good life (virtue) in the US is culturally Christian even in a secular practice.

Throughout this book, we will see how CrossFit does an exceptional job at tapping into several American narratives that give it particular purchase in the lives of those who do it. It illustrates how CrossFit—a fitness regimen that is painful and challenging, quasi-religious and exclusive, heroic and frontier-like, scientific and apocalyptic—comes to feel and be the way in which Americans can live a good, right, virtuous life.[46]

What's Next

We began this chapter with a May 10, 2015, segment called "King of CrossFit" from a *60 Minutes* episode broadcast on CBS News. It hit on a lot of the topics we will explore in this book, such as that CrossFit (like Glassman) is masculine, alienated, patriotic, and tough and rugged American, setting us up nicely to think about the way exercise can tap into various stories and practices that have become meaningful in American life. In chapter 1, we look at how CrossFit is labeled a cult or a religion run by a bike gang and what this means for the community of devoted followers. In chapter 2, we dive deep into the salvation stories that sell CrossFit and how they link suffering, pain, and redemption, which is both a classic American and a Christian story. In chapter 3, we examine the way Greg Glassman operated as an oracle to sell the CrossFit brand and his forging of a revolution in his garage gym. These are time-tested American capitalism myths of the American Dream. In chapter 4, we see the way CrossFit mobilizes old-school tropes of the frontier, including those associated with the US military, special forces, and Manifest Destiny. In chapter 5, we examine the American superhero and the way Christian tropes shape what it means to be heroic. In chapter 6, we spend time with the way science is mobilized by CrossFit, often in scientifically unsound ways. By marshaling frameworks of scientific expertise, CrossFit is trying to appear exceptional as a method of exercise. In chapter 7, we examine the apocalypse as ubiquitous to

American culture and CrossFit. We will see how the COVID-19 pandemic was not the apocalypse that CrossFitters trained for and what that meant during the "end times" of the company and its founder in 2020. In chapter 8, we conclude with an investigation into what is next, for CrossFit and the United States at this cultural moment. While this book is an academic one, I hope nonacademics will also read it, finding each of these elements in the chapters to come, helping us all make sense of the American phenomenon that is CrossFit.

It may seem like we have a lot to get through, and we do. But if you've picked up this book on CrossFit, I imagine you're up for it. So, lace up your shoes, find your spot: "3 . . . 2 . . . 1 . . . Go!"

1

A Cult, a Community, a Religion Run by a Biker Gang

We get asked all the time, "Is this a cult?" And we just get pissed off and say, "No, it's not a cult!" But we heard it so many times and it was asked sincerely enough that it became important to ask the question ourselves: "What if we are a cult I'm running and I don't even know it?" That'd be like the worst kind of cult, right? No, this is an active, loving, sweating, breeding community. Yeah, the caveman thing. I'll tell you what: I don't think it's an insult to any CrossFitter. Yeah, "Cult of the Caveman." What are you going to do?
—Greg Glassman, CrossFit cofounder

"One. Of. Us! One. Of. Us!" the white male CrossFit coach chants. I stop lacing up my new Reebok CrossFit lifting shoes, and I look up to see to whom he is referring. It is me. He has walked up to me as he chants. I look down at my shoes. They are the cheapest ones I could find; lifting shoes are expensive if you are not used to buying specialized sport footwear. Preferring dark shoes, I found my new lifters ugly: all white except for a bit of pink on the soles and "CrossFit" written on the side. But after a few weeks lifting in my running shoes, I had realized I needed to buy lifting shoes for my CrossFit research. You can't lift as heavy in cushiony running shoes.

We make eye contact, and the coach smiles and laughs. His chanting is part teasing—I am not really one of them; I'm an anthropologist studying them. But I am leaning into the "CrossFit lifestyle" by purchasing the CrossFit-labeled shoes.[1] He calls this out in front of everyone. "Soon you'll be drinking the Kool-Aid," he tells me as I stand up, ready for squats. I laugh, one of those break-the-tension laughs, and think, Am I really one of them? What does it mean to be "one of them"? Do I have to "drink the Kool-Aid" to be so? And what does that even really mean?

"Drinking the Kool-Aid" is a common refrain in the United States and in CrossFit. It refers to Jim Jones and Jonestown. Jim Jones was a

Pentecostal pastor, ordained by the Disciples of Christ. He moved his church and congregation, the Peoples Temple of the Disciples of Christ, from California to Guyana, establishing Jonestown. In 1978, the members drank "Kool-Aid" in a mass suicide event (the drink, which was actually a generic flavored drink, was laced with cyanide).[2] "Drinking the Kool-Aid" explicitly indexes dangerous, cult-like devotion and groupthink. It also implicitly indexes Christian death: the suicide at Jonestown and drinking the blood of Christ (Protestant churches in the US use red-colored liquid or grape juice to represent the blood of Christ).[3] The phrase is often used with derision to mean that people are blindly following a leader or beliefs. However, in this case, as is the case with many CrossFitters, it was used with approval and admiration, a reclamation of cult, death, suicide, and Christian references. I was on my way to being "one of them" by purchasing CrossFit paraphernalia. The logical next step was drinking the Kool-Aid.

God's Workout

Before I began my research, I thought that mainstream exercise, health, and nutrition frameworks would shape CrossFit. A common gym narrative in the US is "on and off the bandwagon." Gym-goers get excited and get into a routine "on the bandwagon" (say, as a New Year's resolution), and then they "fall off the bandwagon" when other parts of their life take priority. Then they recommit and get back on the wagon, only to cycle off once more. This is like "yo-yo" dieting. While some people quit CrossFit during my research, most people were fervently devoted to the classes, the community, and the "paleo" diet. They did not regularly fall off just to get back on the bandwagon. They were committed. I heard people talking about apocalypse training, being saved, drinking the Kool-Aid, and CrossFit being a "good cult."[4]

In a 2005 *New York Times* article titled "Getting Fit, Even If It Kills You," Stephanie Cooperman interviewed early adopters of CrossFit: "Mr. Glassman's followers call him Coach and share a cultlike devotion to his theories. . . . 'We are all drinking the Kool-Aid,' said Eugene Allen, another Tacoma SWAT team member. 'It's hard not to catch Coach's enthusiasm.'"[5]

A short few years after the CrossFit website was established, the framework of cult, devotion, and drinking of the Kool-Aid were part of the CrossFit lexicon and framework. Glassman called it a "religion run by a biker gang."[6] Three years later, Virginia Hefferman wrote in the *New York Times Magazine* that CrossFit has "chapters" and a "Book of Common Prayer" and that the CrossFit website is the foundation of a "CrossFit ministry." In the article, titled "God's Workout," Hefferman refers to CrossFitters as "disciples" and describes the program's "cult-like vibe."[7] In 2014, Sean Gregory wrote in *Time*, "CrossFitters admit they can get a little evangelical about their obsession. Says Joshua Newman, a co-owner of CrossFit NYC: 'Are we the Jehovah's Witnesses of exercise? Sure, that's a fair tag.'"

In addition to journalists, divinity students and Christian pastors are also interested in the links between CrossFit and religiosity. In a master's thesis project for Harvard Divinity School, Casper ter Kuile and Angie Thurston investigated ways people gather outside of churches, to understand what constitutes religion and religiosity in the US today.[8] They hosted Glassman at the Divinity School to discuss the links between the exercise regimen and religion.[9] The journalist Michael Schulson flips the narrative on its head and writes of the "CrossFit-ification of Christianity" in the United States:

> The fascinating thing about CrossFit is not that it looks vaguely religious. It's that religion in the United States—in particular, certain strains of Protestant Christianity—is starting to look a lot like CrossFit. "Across the country, congregations are whipping members into shape with highly marketed, faith-based health programs," wrote Leslie Leyland Fields in a *Christianity Today* feature last year.[10] Churches are adding weight rooms and launching weight-loss programs. There's even a consulting firm that specializes in helping churches open gyms.[11]

At One Church in Ohio, Sunday Service is a CrossFit workout.[12]

These American journalists and CrossFitters alike are trying to make sense of CrossFit: its exercise regimen, its frameworks, the devotion people feel to it, and how it reflects American Christian values. Why do participants talk about drinking the Kool-Aid? Why are churches and divinity schools including CrossFit in their services and curricula? Why do people find Glassman to be a fervent "religious" leader with "disciples" and his affiliates to be "chapters"? Why is this exercise method being discussed using Christian terms?

If you have been around a person who identifies as a CrossFitter (which is different from someone who just does CrossFit), you know the deep meaning they give to their commitment, regimen, community, and gym. There are jokes and memes about CrossFitters always talking about CrossFit, which has been referred to as proselytizing: "The gym jock proselytizing at you about CrossFit is a staple cultural stereotype: part braggart, part evangelist, part sentient muscle."[13] Why? Madeline Ulrich writes, "One thing a lot of people don't understand is how hard it is to not talk about something that is a huge part of your life. Somehow everything goes back to CrossFit when you do CrossFit."[14] "Proselytizing" means trying to convert someone. An "evangelist" is someone sharing the "good news," which leads to others converting to Christianity. These terms are used nonchalantly to refer to the way CrossFitters talk about CrossFit. This framing gives CrossFit a meaning well beyond that of simply exercise.

In David Chidester's book, mentioned earlier, *Authentic Fakes: Religion and American Popular Culture*, he examines the "religious dimensions and dynamics of popular culture."[15] He argues that there are a variety of nonreligious cultural activities that do "religious work." For example, he argues that Coca-Cola, Disney, and baseball operate as "fake" religions, but they do "authentic" religious work. That "authentic" religious work is "forging a community, focusing on desire, and facilitating exchange in ways that look just like a religion" without being formally religious.[16]

Chidester argues that popular culture mobilizes the religious techniques of creating sacred time (continuity with the past) and sacred space (location of the sacred) that generate a sense of community within a diverse array of cultural enterprises. Chidester gives the example of "the church of baseball," complete with its own hall of fame that tells the sport's history, or what is commonly referred to as "baseball's mecca." The "meccanization," Chidester calls it, invokes sacredness and helps to cultivate pilgrimages to this "authentically fake" religious space.[17] Cody Musselman illustrates how this works in CrossFit. She examines what she calls "evangelical time," a sacred time associated with "undercurrents of urgency, striving, and the sense of impending doom that exist in American culture" and that reflect "the dynamics of evangelical premillennialism."[18] The sacred space can be found at the annual CrossFit Games, where many CrossFitters make a pilgrimage to watch their favorite elite athletes perform seemingly superhuman capacities, or at the Reebok Fitness Center, where CrossFit coaches "internalize the metaphysics of CrossFit" throughout CrossFit's "be more human" campaign, a campaign, Musselman argues, that links religious frameworks with sport.[19]

Popular culture's religious work is also to focus desire on material objects or commodities in the market economy. Investing sacred meaning in consumer objects has led to them being fetishized, such as the devotion to Apple products or CrossFitters' devotion to CrossFit gear, like the shoes I purchased, which meant that I had been converted. This could also mean turning the body or life into an object that can be realized through consumptive practices. CrossFit muscles are forged through consumptive practices, such as CrossFit gym memberships, grocery store purchases (to follow CrossFit diets), or gear to facilitate improved performance in the workouts; Musselman argues that this is a metaphysical call to be more than human, as in the Reebok "Be More Human Challenge."[20]

(Christian) Fitness Histories

Physical culture practices, exercise strategies, and body politics in the US have a history soaked and cloaked in Christianity. The more overtly Christian ones include, but are certainly not limited to, New Thought or Christian Science circles that focus on fasting and diet, as well as a push to masculinize Christianity and churches through sport in the Muscular Christianity and the YMCA movements.[21] "Serving God could be one effect of exercise, claimed Protestants who were some of the earliest American exercise enthusiasts."[22] Other movements were less overtly Christian but tapped into national frameworks of ideal citizen-subjects that implicitly mobilized Christian terms.[23] One was the move by US presidents and the US government to link ideal national citizenry—complete with frameworks of westward expansion, global dominance, and militarism—with fitness beginning in the 1950s. Another is contemporary fitness culture, with its multibillion-dollar industry, linking morality and "goodness" with exercise and slenderness.[24] Historians have charted these movements, practices, and processes and provided context within which we can understand CrossFit.[25]

One of the most significant investigations into the relationship between Christianity and fitness and diet and the legacies of that relationship is found in the humanities scholar Marie Griffith's *Born Again Bodies*.[26] Griffith illustrates how the culture of Christian fitness appears secular but has deep ties to moral codes and understandings of sin and salvation. She argues, "While Christianity is by no means the only religious tradition able to contribute [to body politics], Protestantism—as the tradition that has most comprehensively influenced the course of American history—takes center stage."[27] New Thought, an American Protestant religious movement beginning in the late 1800s that focused on mind-over-matter thinking, takes a primary focus in her text. New Thought explicitly links corporeality and spirituality, arguing that salvation is found in the body—through health, diet, fasting, sexual restraint, and fitness regimens. Griffith concludes her book by stating, "Modern fitness may not be a 'religion' in the scholarly sense, but it surely has dense and unavoidable religious roots."[28]

One of these roots is the narrative template of mind-over-matter thinking. Early physical culturalists and exercise gurus, like Bernarr Macfadden and Jack LaLanne, were significantly influenced by New Thought ideas. Jonathan Black writes in his book on fitness history, *Making the American Body*, "The term physical culture had been popularized by the world's greatest bodybuilder [Bernarr Macfadden] and dated back to the nineteenth century, its provenance owed to a rediscovery of the body and a rebellion against Victorian restraint. In the twentieth century, it gathered a new momentum in the military, in schools, even in churches, fusing exercise with health and even spirituality."[29]

The title of the first chapter of Macfadden's book (coauthored with Felix Oswald) on the benefits of exercise and fasting asked an evangelical question, "What shall we do to be saved?"[30] Similarly, Jack LaLanne is most famous for his thirty-four-year televised exercise program, for his claim that nutrition and physical culture were "the salvation of America," and for being the "spiritual father of the US fitness movement."[31] These "fathers" followed New Thought ideas and understood American salvation to be linked to body worship and American Christian theology.[32] "While by no means did all New Thought proponents write extensively about physical fitness, enough of them did to affirm this as a chief concern within the movement, albeit one often overlooked by its historians. Rereading New Thought in this way illustrates its vital centrality in the wider American story of dietary and body obsessions."[33]

At the same time that muscled men were preaching New Thought ideas about salvation through proper nutrition and exercise, mainstream Protestant pastors and leaders, including the evangelist and capitalist Dwight L. Moody, President Teddy Roosevelt, and the psychologist / seminary dropout G. Stanley Hall, touted competitive sports and physical education. These Christian men established an American version of the English Muscular Christianity movement. Muscular Christianity is "defined as a Christian commitment to health and manliness," a push to halt what many male leaders thought was the feminization of American Christianity.[34] The Muscular Christianity movement was made popular in the newly institutionalized Young Men's Christian Associations (YMCAs), which were decked out with fitness equipment.[35] Macfadden and LaLanne's New Thought ideas about nutrition, fasting, exercise, and restraint as leading to salvation remain wildly popular among contemporary American fitness folks.[36] Muscular Christianity has transformed into contemporary Christian manliness and sports movements such as the Promise Keepers and the Fellowship of Christian Athletes.[37] CrossFit builds on the link between fitness, the body, and seeking salvation and is seen to be a training for life.[38]

There is a whole faction of CrossFit devoted to Christianity. One of the most famous CrossFit stars is Rich Froning. Froning has won the CrossFit Games, the annual CrossFit international competition, individually or as a member of a team every year since 2011. He proudly claims his devotion to Christianity.[39] His home gym established "CrossFit Faith," which includes Bible study and Christian-informed fitness.[40] This "testimony" and "love of the Lord" inspired others, including Becky Conzelman, who established FAITH RXD, a Christian-based organization linking fitness and a "Christ-centered" life. FAITH RXD is a mission that leads to "Chapters," or "volunteer-led groups that strengthen fitness affiliate owners, coaches, and athletes for Christ-centered living and impact through workouts, faith-based discussion, prayer, social and service events. . . . Chapters meet every month, *all over the world in 80+ cities in 9 countries.*"[41] In other words, one can easily find an overt Christian CrossFit message. Covert Christian messages or cultural Christian messages also abound.

My research was conducted on the edge of gentrified Brooklyn in an old warehouse. It is filled with progressive, generous people, mostly those who might identify as a "None" in the Pew Research terminology of religious affiliation.[42] The owner could be identified as "Goth" in his all-black outfit, black eyeliner, long dark hair, and a penchant for occult-type paraphernalia. His art adorns the gym and is what he calls "dark" or on the "macabre side."[43] He questions the praying that people do to "the invisible alpha male in the sky," and he believes that the "secular story of our species through biology and evolution manages to be more inspiring, sobering, and liberating than all the worlds [sic] mythologies and superstitions combined."[44] He and his gym surely do not come off as Christian.

But Goth style cannot quite be understood outside of Christian frameworks. Occult imagery demands Christianity for its meaning. This is the way that cultural Christianity works: it is always there, Christian histories sitting in the room already. It becomes attached to innocuous or subversive elements despite secular or anti-Christian consciousnesses. Therefore, the afterlives of Christian values and themes, cultural Christianity, emerged in this Brooklyn gym despite the owner's best efforts to be "Goth" or occult, or as members trained for a "zombie apocalypse" rather than a Christian one. Christian themes and values are there in underlying codes even when we are not really looking for them or when, if we see their opposite, we believe they can't be present.[45] Mostly they sneak in; they are already there to begin with, sitting in the chair in the empty room.

The differences between these two types of gym are significant; places like the Brooklyn CrossFit gym are "secular" compared to FAITH RXD. However, the Christianity that leads to something like FAITH RXD is the same one that leads to devotional adherence to CrossFit gym communities, coaches, ideologies, and practices outside of explicit faith-based organizations. One is soaked in Christianity. The other is cloaked. They look different, but the wake of Christianity shaped the forging of the CrossFit brand, because it, like other aspects of American culture, such as the American work ethic or democracy, includes Christian values. CrossFit pivots among a "cult," "a community," and "a religion run by a biker gang," all as cultural Christian afterlives.

Cults and CrossFit

What is a cult? How did we come to use that word so commonly? The scholar of religion and ethnographer of CrossFit Cody Musselman provides a thorough context:

> The word cult comes from the Latin word *cultus*, meaning to cultivate, grow, or worship. From the seventeenth century onward, it has been used to describe religious sects and or groups that direct their veneration to a particular figure, deity, or object. By the mid-nineteenth century its meaning had expanded to include the adoration of non-religious things, like the "cult of success." Its meaning further evolved during the mid-to-late twentieth century during a boom in alternative religions and new religious and spiritual organizations, and "cult" became a pejorative label used to describe and denigrate fringe religious groups. At first, in the 1950s and 1960s, cults were thought of as anomalous and largely harmless oddities. From the 1970s onward, however, the notion that cults were dangerous and housed social deviants increased. During the heyday of the cult controversies in the 1970s and 1980s, being accused of membership in a cult was decidedly bad, and anti-cult groups like Ted Patrick's FREECOG and "cult deprogrammers" emerged to manage the public concern around cults. The fear of cults intensified with media coverage of sensational and sometimes violent events such as the Manson Family murders in 1969, the mass suicides of the People's Temple at Jonestown in 1978, Heaven's Gate in 1997, and the stand-off between federal agents and the Branch Davidians in Waco, TX, in 1993.[46]

Cult designations are contrasted with mainline religion, often set in binary terms: good versus bad religion. Good religion usually means mainline Protestant in the United States. Bad is a group like the Peoples Temple.[47] Being designated a cult can mean being tagged as a "dangerous pseudo-religion with satanic overtones" that leads to the physical, sexual, and economic exploitation of members by a charismatic, brainwashing leader.[48] To label a movement a cult is to suggest that it is not the kind of religion that benefits society or produces good citizens. The "cult" label even goes so far as to suggest that the movement is not a religion at all. In 1993, the political scientist Michael Barkun wrote that to "dub a group a 'cult' is to associate it with irrationality and authoritarianism. Its leaders practice 'mind control,' its members have been 'brainwashed' and its beliefs are 'delusions.' To be called a 'cult' is to be linked not to religion but to psychopathology."[49] No wonder Greg Glassman did not want CrossFit to be called a cult in the epigraph to this chapter.

But by the 2000s, popular culture would transform the term, include it as a punch line rather than a threat, or rebrand it as something economically advantageous. "Cult" became a brand strategy.[50] Douglas Atkin, the global head of community for Airbnb, claims in his 2004 book *The Culting of Brands* that cults are a *"good thing," "normal,"* and that "people join them for *very good reasons.*"[51] Cult brands are supposed to tap into people's desires to express their individuality while belonging to a community, a feeling of being outside the status quo and exclusionary.[52] Musselman writes that this contrarian, exclusive group and its identity formation are "perhaps what makes CrossFit most appear like a cult to outside observers and insiders alike."[53] Musselman contextualizes the label of CrossFit as a cult. It has a zealous founder and leader (Glassman), who established the regimen in opposition to mainstream gyms, with their typical exercisers (people on rows of ellipticals watching television through headphones) and a business strategy of having many members who do not show up. CrossFitters themselves evangelize the good news of CrossFit and proselytize to get anyone and everyone to try it. Musselman uses the classic CrossFit joke: "A vegan, an atheist, and a CrossFitter walk into a bar. You know because they tell you."[54]

Due to the affiliate model (the model CrossFit uses to allow certified CrossFit coaches to open their own CrossFit gyms, which includes an application and small annual fee, rather than a franchise model, in which all gyms look the same), people could find a CrossFit box that mirrored their own identity—a conservative Christian CrossFit, a veteran-owned and military-infused CrossFit, a LGBTQ+-friendly CrossFit, and so on—thereby linking identity to community and individual box to Cross-

Fit writ large. This process mirrors the sectarian nature of American Protestant Christian congregational churches, in which the congregations make the rules of the church, not the Catholic pope, and they all can fit nicely under the umbrella of Protestant Christianity. CrossFit gyms are able to be both their local flavor and identified with a larger brand, business, or movement.

Using interviews with CrossFit personalities and a CrossFit discussion board questionnaire, Musselman examines how participants explained the cult-like culture of CrossFit: CrossFitters have their own special language; they follow a special diet; they all get T-shirts from other CrossFit gyms and wear them proudly; they have a special meeting place, the gym; they follow a zealous leader; any kind of resistance is discouraged or punished; the group is elitist, believing it has an exalted status; there is an "us-versus-them" mentality; guilt and shame are used as motivating strategies; there is a proselytizing mission to recruit more members; and "true believers" feel that there is no life outside of the group.[55] When Glassman was asked to respond to the question of whether CrossFit is a cult, he responded in part with the quotation in the epigraph to this chapter, a shrug, and a "What are you going to do?" as if being called a cult was not so bad and was not entirely inaccurate. But he did not design CrossFit to be a cult; it just filled a need in people: "The magic is in the movement, the art is in the programming, the science is in the explanation, and the fun is in the community."[56] Because, ultimately, CrossFit is not about training for a sport or going to the gym to zone out for an hour on an elliptical; rather, it is training for life in a fun-loving community.

CVFM @HI + Communal Environment = Health

In a beautifully produced video I found on New Orleans's CrossFit Full Bore South's website, titled "What Is CrossFit in Six Words?," the equation setting of this section is explained.[57] It is one of a few official definitions of CrossFit. The six-word phrase is common knowledge in CrossFit: "constantly varied functional movement at high intensity," or "CVFM@HI." Glassman added the "+ Communal Environment = Health" later, completing the formula for CrossFit's success. Let us take each in turn.

"CV" means "constantly varied." One of the cornerstones of CrossFit is that the workouts always change, preparing participants for the all the unknown situations that life throws at people. "FM" means "functional movement," or exercises resembling natural, everyday activities rather than exercises only found at a gym (e.g., squats help you stand up from a chair, rather than knee extensions on a seated machine at the gym, which are simply about muscle development). "@HI" means at "at high intensity," referring to the workouts being challenging, difficult, painful, and requiring pushing through one's limits. This contrasts with being able to get on an elliptical machine and get lost in a television show while exercising. Finally, the "+ Communal Environment," which Glassman added later, after the regimen was established and CrossFit became synonymous with group fitness at the fifteen thousand gyms worldwide, means doing it with others, in a class, with people you see every day at 6 a.m. or 5 p.m. or with people at the CrossFit gym you drop into in, say, Cusco, Peru; Marrakesh, Morocco; or Hong Kong. When I began my research on CrossFit, everyone would reference "the community" as a meaningful part of their experience of the exercise regimen.

To try to understand the CrossFit community alchemic process, journalists have examined CrossFit, and academics have conducted studies, written papers, and published books.[58] There are several ways to parse what people mean by "community." Perhaps CrossFit is what the sociologist Ray Oldenburg termed a "third space"—a place not home or work—where people go and make connections and establish bonds?[59] This is true, but the bonds seem deeper, cosmic, and metaphysical, rather than interpersonal. Maybe the CrossFit community is organized on what the social and community psychologist Seymour Sarason defined as a sense of community (SOC), or the feeling that one is part of a readily available, supportive, and dependable structure.[60] Scholars of recreation, sport management, and kinesiology used the "sense of community" to investigate CrossFit participation as compared to other group and individual fitness activities.[61] Another sport-science paper investigates the success of CrossFit in bringing high-intensity training (usually associated with the military or elite athletics) to the general population. The authors write, "There is a strong sense of community within CrossFit and new participants are expected to 'buy-into' this culture. CrossFitters are expected to support and encourage each other and attend on a regular basis."[62]

As an anthropologist, I have sought definitions of "community" in our literature; many anthropologists have studied "communitas," or a transformational element central to rites of passage. "Communitas" was coined by the anthropologist of religion Victor Turner, who defined the structural elements of ritual and argued that ritual is the experience of liminality—when the usual rules of daily life are suspended or inverted—in a group setting.[63] The anthropologist Edith Turner (Victor Turner's wife) further enhanced his definition of "communitas," arguing that liminality's communitas is "inspired fellowship or collective joy."[64] But liminality, rites of passage, and the communitas therein are not daily occurrences but once-in-a-lifetime ritual events.

The Harvard divinity students Angie Thurston and Casper ter Kuile pushed these frameworks of community further by examining "how American millennials gather." Seventy-two percent of Nones (Americans who do not claim a religion in Pew research studies) are under the age of fifty, a similar demographic to CrossFit gyms. To understand why younger Americans do not affiliate with any religion, Thurston and ter Kuile conducted research on various ways millennials "gather" or seek meaning and find community in nonchurch spaces. They focused on ten spaces of social gathering for younger people, including CrossFit, the "dinner party," and social justice projects. They analyzed these ten case studies of spaces of gathering, which tapped into Christian or religious themes such as community, personal transformation, social transformation, purpose, creativity, and accountability. They argue that CrossFit provides community, personal transformation, and accountability and does so with "evangelical enthusiasm."[65]

Thurston and ter Kuile's master's thesis was the reason Harvard Divinity School asked CrossFit creator Greg Glassman to come and speak to students about his (and CrossFit's) mission. Glassman recounts that he had a conversation with an army captain and Green Beret, Michael Perry. Perry attested that camaraderie in special forces is fundamental, as it is in CrossFit. The defining elements of that camaraderie, according to Perry, are "agony and laughter." Glassman maintains that coaches and owners of CrossFit gyms "get to" blur traditional boundaries between professionals and clients and become friends, lovers, or partners. This close bonding encourages "agony and laughter" in a physical pursuit and becomes the foundation of the CrossFit community.[66] Glassman states that people in CrossFit are having both the best and the worst times of their lives, and "that does something very different to you."⁶⁷ But he does not say what that something is. I think the answer can be found in Josiah Royce's beloved community.

The phrase "beloved community" is often, and rightly, associated with the Reverend Dr. Martin Luther King Jr. in his pursuit of racial justice through nonviolence in the US during the 1960s. However, the phrase's origin is in late-1800s American philosophical thought. "Beloved community" was coined by the philosopher Josiah Royce in a series of lectures and texts published in the early 1900s. Royce was born in California in 1855 to English immigrants who sought a new beginning in the American West as pioneers on the edge of the frontier.⁶⁸ His upbringing in the American frontier undoubtedly shaped his understanding of the significance of social life in one's finding a "central aim" in one's life.⁶⁹ Social processes "established a way of life, instilled values, and pursued ethical causes," giving meaning and coherence to "the self."⁷⁰ In 1899, Royce would argue that "to be" (the quintessential philosophical question) was to be uniquely oneself while being in relation to a whole.⁷¹ In other words, it was participation in a beloved community that would orient and give meaning to individuals.

Royce's beloved community is forged through a particular form of loyalty: "By loyalty I mean the *practically devoted love of an individual for a community*."⁷² These communities could be family, home, village, tribe, clan, or country.⁷³ Or CrossFit. This kind of community provides what Royce identifies as loyalty that inspires faith, attachment, and devotion to it. Royce does not equate this faith and attachment with something mystical but rather with the practicality of those who want to be a good friend, citizen, or home-loving being. This is not the same loyalty we find in marriage or the military but "the willing and thoroughgoing devotion of a self to a cause, when the cause is something which unites many selves in one, and which is therefore the interest of a community."⁷⁴ This community is *superior* to the selves that form it, more *real* than the selves in it.⁷⁵ This beloved community forged on communitarian love is seen in the Apostle Paul's version of Christianity (Pauline) and was made popular by Dr. King. But Royce believed that the beloved community is not some fanciful dream, a wishful Pollyanna-ism, but a "real, achievable, concrete community of heaven and earth."[76] It does not just happen, though; it has to be created.

While the beloved community is understood by Royce and King as a Christian entity, it is also the kind of community that, I argue, CrossFit is. CrossFit is forged and maintained by a practical, devoted love of an individual for a community. Many adherents take on the name CrossFitter as a form of self-identity, but this self-identity is forged in a "beloved community" in which people find meaning in their membership and in which the community is searching for deep meaning and salvation together.

Biker Gangs, *Fight Club*, Beloved Community?

Miranda Joseph argues in her book *Against the Romance of Community* that too often in the United States, "community" carries with it only positive notions and obscures existing stressors in these collectives. Joseph argues that a shared single "identity" is the bond that establishes community, and this single-identity-based community conceals other identities that might be in tension with the dominant one.[77] CrossFitters are known for the positive features of their collective identity, but other characteristics of the "CrossFit community" reveal some negative connotations of the collective as well. The mobilization of "a religion run by a biker gang" and *Fight Club* reflects some of the not-so-positive elements of loyalty and identity-from-community, including racially motivated forms of exclusion and glorified masculine violence.

The "biker gang" that I think Glassman is referring to is the Hells Angels, a California motorcycle club.[78] According to their own lore, the Hells Angels are a group of rebellious, violent white men who are often veterans living on the edges of society, alienated from mainstream culture due to shifts in capitalist structures and notions of normative masculinity.[79] They are often portrayed as a racially and gendered homogeneous group (white men only) with a chip on their shoulder and charter clubs.[80] While CrossFit is not male only, its ethos is based on toughness, dominance, and in-your-face intensity, or as scholars have defined this ethos, "hegemonic masculinity."[81] Glassman thinks the CrossFit community is organized on "agony and laughter" like the Green Berets, a special forces group that did not allow women until 2020 and would still prefer that they not join.[82] The biker gang and agony and laughter valorize a tough, in-your-face masculinity that has colored CrossFit regardless of CrossFitters' gender identity.

The Hells Angels come with their own fierce-looking mascot: a white skull as a face and yellow and red wings for hair. It screams, "Don't mess with us." CrossFit's own mascot resembles the Hells Angels one. Pukey the Clown (also known as Uncle Rhabdo) is a fierce-looking white-faced clown with long yellow or orange hair flowing from each temple. Pukey is puking and Uncle Rhabdo is bleeding and hooked up to a dialysis machine (treatment for rhabdomyolisis) because puking and bleeding after a CrossFit workout is both a rite of passage and a common occurrence for the hard-core participants.[83] These mascots are both caricature (Glassman says that the clown is funny) and stark reminder that CrossFit, when done correctly, can cause puking, bleeding, or organ failure. Glassman says that CrossFit can kill you, and he has been completely honest about that reality.[84] It does not get more valorizing of tough or hegemonic masculinity than to participate in a workout that can kill you when you push yourself too hard.

These images and references to self-induced bleeding and puking link CrossFit to another countercultural group in popular culture that emerged right before CrossFit. *Fight Club*, the novel and film, has found not only critical acclaim but a "cult" following in the 1990s.[85] For characters, readers, and viewers, fight club was a radical response to the alienation that white men were feeling at the end of the twentieth century's late-stage capitalism.[86] They had been "feminized" by going to college and by consumer culture and, therefore, were in desperate need of masculine violence to feel alive. Chuck Palahniuk writes in *Fight Club*, "You aren't alive anywhere like you're alive in fight club. . . . You see a guy come to fight club for the first time, and his ass is a loaf of white bread. You see this same guy here six months later, and he looks carved out of wood. . . . There's grunting and noise at fight club like at the gym, but fight club isn't about looking good. There's hysterical shouting in tongues like at church, and when you wake up Sunday afternoon you feel saved."[87] One could replace fight club with CrossFit, and it would ring true to the ideals of the workout regimen. Sure, fight club is hand-to-hand combat, and CrossFit is a workout. But in both, the feeling of being alive comes from the rigors of a bloody physical pursuit. One arrives as a "loaf of white bread" and after six months is "carved out of wood"; the grunting and noise resound like speaking in tongues at a church, where you wake up from a fight/workout feeling saved. As noted earlier, the overwhelming majority of CrossFitters are white, and despite equal numbers of women and men, the regimen is built on hegemonic masculine ideals of violence and toughness.

Perhaps CrossFit is a community of alienated, rebellious, masculine, mostly white followers who feel seen by the countercultural framework of the group.[88] The camaraderie is built in the self-violence and agony of the workouts as well as a community of like-minded individuals who feel more whole through their participation in CrossFit. The beloved community is not like King's, which is about racial justice and social equity, but it is "beloved" in Royce's sense of loyalty to the group as quintessential for the identity of the participant. It is a beloved community, which through various pop-culture references and whether participants consciously ascribe to those values or not, is forged on self-violent hegemonic masculinity and white alienation.

Conclusion

Despite the equation CVFM@HI + Communal Environment = Health, CrossFit workouts are not only about health. Much like other fitness practices, diet, exercise, and health, CrossFit is linked in the United States to Christian frameworks: the early famous physical culturalists providing salvation through commitment to better body practices. CrossFit is a contemporary version of fitness that is linked to "religion" or Christianity. In other words, cultivating "religious" meaning in exercise is not revolutionary; it has been common, historically. However, being identified as a cult is new; it is linked to changes in historical uses of the term, including in marketing and capitalism. Therefore, people take on the otherwise pejorative frameworks of "cult" or "Kool-Aid drinker" because CrossFit emerged in a time when to do so made sense to a large, devoted following of people who were "all in." CrossFit feels cultish because it taps into culturally Christian afterlives that Americans do not even realize are Christian and because the term "cult" has taken on a different meaning in today's capitalist landscape. I argue that CrossFit is a beloved community, building on the framework of "loyalty" in the work of the frontier philosopher Josiah Royce. The beloved community is forged on a loyalty to something beyond oneself, where the self is fashioned in communally prescribed ways including self-violent masculinity and white alienation. The practice that does this is painful, supportive group exercising that ultimately combines agony and laughter, a community of sufferers, as we will discuss in chapter 2. I think when Glassman says that CrossFit "does something to you," he means that it *saves* you. CrossFit is a beloved community, and it is through this beloved community that one finds salvation.

2

Salvation through Bearing One's Daily Cross(Fit)

Then he said to them all: "Whoever wants to be my disciple must deny themselves and take up their cross daily and follow me. For whoever wants to save their life will lose it, but whoever loses their life for me will save it."
—Luke 9:23–24

Go to any CrossFit gym's website and you will find testimonials. The testimonials sell the gym: the CrossFit regimen, the knowledgeable coaches, and the fun community. They have a typical structure: tales of fear or uncertainty about CrossFit but needing an exercise regimen, trying CrossFit, and being transformed from the experience. A white woman in the Mountain West whom I call Kelsey writes on her CrossFit gym's webpage, "I can honestly say that walking in those doors is one of the best decisions I have ever made!" Those who visit the gym's website and read the testimonials might be inspired to give it a try, hoping for the same experience as those who inspired them, hoping that walking through the doors of CrossFit might also be one of the best decisions of their lives.

We begin our exploration of how salvation works in the CrossFit gym for the mostly white Americans who participate in it with a testimonial from a white woman living in the Midwest whom I call Rachel. Other CrossFitters' stories will follow. These emblematic examples illustrate the stories people tell, the feelings people feel, and the communities people build on these stories and feelings. All of them are illustrative of the active ingredients of CrossFit salvation. It is no coincidence that this salvation mirrors Christian salvation.

We will focus on three key elements in CrossFit salvation. First, one must try it: "walk through the doors" of the gym. This sounds simple enough. But due to CrossFit lore, sometimes people are fearful or apprehensive to give it a try. Second, the workout must be challenging and painful. CrossFit is known for its intense, painful workouts. Enter any CrossFit gym at the end of an hour, and you will see CrossFitters sprawled out on the floor, destroyed from the workout, arms perpendicular to the body, like Christ on the cross. CrossFitters must push themselves to painful limits and find meaning in this part of the practice. If you do not, you are not really doing it correctly. Third, one must make friends or find community to sustain the challenge and pain of the workouts. Theoretically, one can do the workouts alone, but CrossFit is done in a class setting, which is a major draw of the regimen. CrossFitters are known for encouraging one another: cheering, high fives, and circling around watching each other finish. They push one another along with what is known in CrossFit as "healthy competition." People become regulars—6 a.m.-ers, 5 p.m.-ers—and this allows for daily interactions with the same people. These daily interactions allow people to become close, build bonds, and share intimacies such as diet changes, strength gains, and recovery or rest strategies. Soon people tend to see "results," such as muscles in places they did not have before, lost inches around the waist, friends to hang out with after class, and just feeling like a part of something. These "results" encourage people to commit to exercise in ways they have not ever done before. The challenging regimen, the camaraderie, the physical changes are really meaningful and come to feel really good. People keep coming back. All of these elements become part of someone's transformation or salvation through CrossFit. They are asked to write about why they keep coming back and "what CrossFit means to them" for the gym's website, exhorting others on the fence or new to the area to come and see what CrossFit is about. These testimonials of redemption through the practice and community of CrossFit are the "good news," gospel, message of salvation of CrossFit.

The public declarations of finding purpose and being saved have deep roots in Christianity, notably with Augustine's *Confessions* in 401 CE.[1] For Augustine, the name "confessions" isn't just about confessing one's faith but also refers to all kinds of religiously authorized speech.[2] Confessions of faith are formal statements of doctrinal belief ordinarily intended for public avowal by an individual, a group, a congregation, a synod, or a church; confessions are like creeds, although usually more extensive. They are particularly associated with the churches of the Protestant Reformation in Europe, with white Christian churches in the US, and with the destiny of the US nation-state more generally.[3] Christian testimonies emerge in the wake of this history, and an individual's "confession of faith" takes a particular narrative arc: one's life before meeting Christ, how one knew one needed Christ and acknowledged that, and one's life after meeting Christ.[4] This is not just about Augustine's *Confessions*, however. Narratives of redemption can be found throughout US history, and they either include personal experience and autobiographical accounts of conversion or are a reshaping of everyday life in the context of a community.[5] American CrossFit follows both.

Swap CrossFit for God or Christ or church, and Rachel's testimony below follows this script and narrative arc. What one's life was like before CrossFit (bad), how one found CrossFit, and how life has been after joining CrossFit (good). The story is one with trackable "sins" in both the Christian and CrossFit traditions, for example, gluttony. Then there is a revelation that the old way of life is somehow wrong, bad, or unsustainable. Finally, a way out is revealed, a path to redemption and salvation through a commitment to CrossFit and the life this commitment provides. I share Rachel's entire testimonial here. She has organized her testimonial into sections. I have italicized key sentences throughout and will return to them at the end. But as you will notice, much like the biblical epigraph to this chapter, Rachel denies herself and takes up her daily "Cross"(Fit) and in so doing becomes a disciple who loses her life and is saved.

Rachel's Testimony

I have gone through just about every exercise phase and craze there is: Running, Swimming, Les Mills programs (Body Pump, RPM, etc.), Kickboxing, Yoga, Personal Strength Training, and, at one point, I was even a certified spin instructor: I was never an athlete. I only played sports to be social in high school, but I have always loved exercise, specifically group exercise. While I am able to motivate myself more than most to work out on my own, a group setting has always been my favorite.

As much as I have always loved exercise . . . it is important to note that *I have the worst eating habits . . . ever!* I have eaten like a 12 year old for most of my life as the standard. I love fried foods, sugar, and bread and eat almost no veggies or fruit. In the past, I would try "quick fixes" like crazy diets that are unsustainable or diet pills. *Nothing ever stuck.* I would eat better for a small amount of time, or in the case of the pills, I would just eat less of the crappy food. It would work for a short time *but I would always eventually end up going back to my horrible habits.*

ENTER CROSSFIT [GYM NAME].
When I moved to [midwestern city], I was trying to find something that was going to work with my schedule, budget, and exercise needs. I was able to use the gym at my apartment and I would try to incorporate strength movements from a book but it was miserable and I could only motivate myself to even do anything about half the time. I tried Title Boxing in [midwestern city] because I had done those classes while living in NYC the year before and had loved them, high energy, strength work, and you get to HITT [sic] stuff:) However, I quickly realized with the behemoth that is [midwestern city] traffic, I was never going to be able to have a regular routine there that would work with my schedule.

I had been talking (complaining) to a colleague at my school about my lack of a "good workout" in my area. *He is a CrossFit convert and had actually been promoting it since I met him. I had blown him off and called him a cult member* and all of the regular things you say to someone who does CrossFit. *He finally convinced me to try it. . . .* I told him with as close as I lived to CrossFit [gym name], *I really didn't have an excuse not to at least give it a shot* so I signed up for the free intro. *I was apprehensive to say the least. I had many preconceived notions and judgments about the "type of people" that do CrossFit,* but I went in anyway. I was super up front and had no problems sharing my preconceived notions about how CrossFit people just want to lift a bunch of heavy weight and how it's a fad that gets people hurt because they really don't teach proper form. *By the end of the intro session,* their knowledge of fitness had convinced me to give it a try. *I signed up for the intro month* which allowed me to have a couple of one-on-one sessions to go over the basic movements and then jumped into classes. I still very vividly remember one of the first workouts. I was halfway through a set of burpees on a time limit and *I realized I don't think I had ever been that challenged physically or, if I'm honest, mentally.* I HATE BURPEES! *I seriously questioned what I had gotten into* and for a brief moment wondered *if I was cut out for it* and if I should even come back. . . . Almost 8 months later and I'm still here. . . . Not planning on going anywhere anytime soon :)

I do have to say that, surprisingly, the biggest effect CrossFit [gym name] has had on me is my nutrition. *For the first time in my life*, I realized and felt how much the extra weight I carry was affecting my performance. I think in other areas (spin, swimming, even weight lifting), I was able to perform even at a heavier weight. I remember there was a moment about 3 months in at [CrossFit gym name] that for the first time ever, I thought to myself "I work too damn hard in those workouts to completely negate it by eating so unhealthily." For the first time, *I wanted to eat better so I could perform better, not just to look better.*

ENTER THE WELLNESS CHALLENGE IN JANUARY.
At just the right time, they started advertising for the Wellness Challenge. I was in a different mindset than I had ever been before and *I was ready for something to help guide me*, keep me accountable, and teach me how to eat in order to get my body to perform better. "Winning" wasn't even a consideration for me as I am the least competitive person in the world. The challenge was just a way to utilize others around me and the knowledge that the coaches brought to tap into my desire to be healthier. *The first week was absolutely miserable, but with the help of seeing others' misery* on the Facebook page, and this newfound motivation, *I got through*. I finally felt what it was like to have my body function well. My energy levels were amazing and *I just felt great! I also saw the eating patterns as something I could continue to stick with*, again, for the first time in my life. Eating healthy was totally doable. I ended up losing almost 13 pounds and several inches in 6 weeks which felt GREAT. Also, I won!!! Winning was super cool but was secondary to the life changes that came from the challenge. I am far from perfect but *I am a completely different person in regards to nutrition than I was a year ago*, which is probably the biggest "win" for me.

WHAT CROSSFIT [GYM NAME] MEANS TO ME
I am convert, a Kool-Aid drinker, a cult member, and a lifer. In such a short amount of time, *I have seen my body change, become stronger, function more efficiently, and I am able to do things I never thought I would be able to do*. Every class I take, *I am challenged and pushed to my limit*, causing me to get stronger (literally) every day. I said I am not a competitive person, which is true, but I do compete with myself. I hold myself to high standards and will push to meet those standards. CrossFit gives me something to work for ev-

ery time I step into the gym. I still scale down so many things in work-outs, but I now know what it feels like to push myself.

I would be remiss if I neglected to talk about the impact the CrossFit [gym name] community has had on me. Moving to a new city is never easy and finding a community of like-minded individuals is typically one of the hardest parts. Starting with the Barbellas girls group, and eventually many others in the gym, what I found at CrossFit [gym name] was a *diverse group of individuals that are supportive,* genuinely like being around each other, and all place wellness and fitness as a priority in their lives. How can you not love a group like that?

To sum it up, I would say that *[CrossFit gym name] has given me a supportive community that has helped me make life changes and grow physically and mentally stronger* through putting fitness *and* nutrition as a priority in my life. Not to mention ... CrossFit [gym name] throws killer parties :)

Rachel's story is moving. One can see how she goes from feeling lost to trying CrossFit, even though she was convinced it was not going to be right for her (the regimen or the people). She throws herself into it and experiences various forms of pain and misery. She pushes through these terrible experiences, however, and emerges out of them feeling great, supported, and ready to commit to this cult of other wonderful and committed people.

Rachel's story takes on the classic salvation *Confessions* narrative form but also has the unique combination of American elements, personal insight and conversion, and ongoing life changes within a community. Part of the transformative process for CrossFitters in general and Rachel in particular is the pain and suffering they go through. Salvation, transformation, is not an easy process. Rather, Rachel was pushed to her limits, past what she had been capable of doing in her past, and she hung on. She emerged from this pain and misery a new person, saved from her former bad-habit self. That pain and suffering are part of the process of being saved is critical. Without the pain and suffering, the pushing of limits, and sharing that misery with others, Rachel might not have committed and transformed herself. Why is the pain so important? And why does sharing the misery with others mean so much?

The Suffering and Saved Self

The scholar of religion Ariel Glucklich examines what he calls "sacred pain."[6] Sacred pain is not "an 'unwanted guest'" but "a useful and important sensation worthy of understanding and cultivating." He maintains that "the goal of religious life is not to bring anesthesia, but to transform the pain that causes suffering into a pain that leads to insight, meaning, and even salvation." Glucklich writes that physical suffering stands "at the center of Christian life, beginning with the sacrifice of Christ and running through the capacity to imitate the suffering of Christ." This Christian suffering and pain are "always and mysteriously related to truth," educating people in "patience and perseverance, which are necessary for salvation."[7]

Salvation through Pain and Suffering

Christianity is organized and based on suffering and pain, especially for Christians with European origins or cultivated in the white American traditions.[8] The religious scholar Judith Perkins argues in her book on early Christian narratives that Christianity, through Jesus Christ's focus on engaging with and healing or feeding the poor, sick, hungry, and downtrodden, brought a suffering self and pained body into cultural consciousness. In addition, Christianity as a religion "centers on suffering in the exemplar of the crucified Christ."[9] In other words, Christianity—through Jesus's focus on the pain and suffering of others and his own crucifixion—and early writings about Christ's suffering helped establish a recognizable body and self that suffered.[10] It also includes the pain and suffering of those who were persecuted for their Christian beliefs over the past two thousand years.[11] The German scholar of ancient Christianity and Protestant theology Christoph Markschies writes in a journal focused on the treatment of pain, "Pain and Christianity appear to belong together: Christ's pain stands at the centre of God's healing; his pain leads to the salvation of mankind. We can learn from Jesus' example how to bear suffering and pain. . . . The memory of the fact that Jesus himself had to undergo the worst pain can still help people to overcome their pain and comfort them."[12]

Pain and Christianity belong together. Early Christian writers "gave Christian suffering a privileged position in explaining the impetus behind conversions."[13] Bodily suffering became something to pay attention to and understand, and it "provided Christians with their community identity."[14] Christian pain was "a weapon by means of which the body [was] subdued, demons exorcised, temptations averted, in a battle for salvation."[15] It was only through the pain of workouts and the misery of resisting food temptations that Rachel subdued her body's resistance to "bad habits" and found deliverance.

Christian pain does not end with pain, however; it also includes comfort and healing. Jesus healed the pain and suffering of the sick, poor, and downtrodden. His painful death was the precursor for his resurrection. The pain had to be gone through to emerge healed, transformed, born again. Christianity centers on pain and suffering *and* liberation through pain and suffering. Pain is an alchemic force, "which magically transforms its victim from one state of existence to a higher, purer state."[16] Rachel's liberation comes through her misery; she pushes her limits and sticks with the misery enough to emerge transformed, resurrected, a "completely different person."

Not everyone thinks of pain as good or liberatory.[17] The International Association for the Study of Pain defines pain as "an unpleasant sensory and emotional experience associated with, or resembling that associated with, actual or potential tissue damage."[18] This association was created to bring health practitioners and scientists together to "bring relief to those in pain."[19] Medical anthropologists also investigate pain, focusing on chronic pain and suffering and the ways in which people try to find relief.[20] In this research, rather than pain being self-imposed, it is generally thrust on people through an unwanted medical experience or illness. Pain *relief* is the primary concern of these scholars, not cultivating it as sacred or meaningful.

CrossFit's pain and suffering can be both sacred and chronic. Much like for Christian martyrs, in CrossFit, "It's the experience of pain—not its absence—that signifies the spiritual realm. . . . Pain is not biological but cosmic."[21] As with Rachel, the misery of diet changes and doing burpees, a dynamic exercise in which one moves from standing to a plank to a push-up to a squat, finishing with a jump (which she hates), to push her physical and mental limits is meaningful. They lead to self-transformation: "being a new person" with a "new lifestyle" that centers on misery and pushing limits. And this pushing of limits is habitual. The pain is not part of a once-in-a-lifetime rite of passage or religious pilgrimage but suffered daily, a daily cross(fit). It is chronic, sacred pain.

Marcia's Pain Cave: The Christian Themes of a Nonbeliever

What does it look like to be pushed to one's limit? The "pain cave" is a pervasive metaphor in CrossFit (and other intense sporting endeavors) that illustrates WOD (workout of the day) pain. In popular culture, the "pain cave" "refers to the point in a workout or competition where the activity seems impossibly difficult. . . . In the athlete community, working through the pain cave is seen as a test of mental resilience."[22] The "pain cave" refers to the psychological aspects associated with physical pain, the dangers of an athlete's attitude about the inevitable pain, and the possibilities (fate) of pushing through it.[23] I asked CrossFitters to describe or draw their pain caves.[24] Marcia's is illustrative:

> [The] pain cave has a dark black tunnel leading to it that kind of looks like the inside of a whale stomach. It leads to this big metal door. Inside the pain cave, it's dark, hot, red; getting to this room is scary, dark, ominous. It kind of reminds me of hell. It feels really hard to breathe; I can't think straight. You just hear self-doubt when you're in this room. Once you're in the room long enough, there is this big, gated metal door and then a wooden door. These lead to the top of a mountain peak where it's quiet and you feel clarity, relief. Like you can breathe. When you get through those rough moments of the pain cave and you feel free after, there's fresh air which represents freedom and growth. Just you and thousands of clouds and the sky around you.

Here we see Marcia make sense of her pain cave through use of Christian imagery found in the King James Bible New Testament. Jesus retells the Old Testament account of Jonah in the "belly of a whale." Christianity provides many interpretations and meanings to the famous "fish" or "whale" and Jonah. But Marcia's use of the "whale belly" here is suggestive of a common one: a terrifying swallowing, three days in the belly of the beast, and then the miraculous emergence of Jonah, alive.[25] Marcia emerges, miraculously, from her pain cave. Marcia notes that the cave explicitly reminds her of hell because it is dark, hot, and red—all reflective of common cultural Christianity's understandings of hell. The idea of doors and movement through them evokes Dante's journey in the *Inferno* of his *Divine Comedy*, including awaking in a dark wood of terror through the gates of hell (the big, gated metal door) and wandering through a dark tunnel past several other (wooden) doors until he makes it to the top of a hill. The emergence out of the inferno/hell and toward paradise and salvation is akin to Marcia's arrival in a heaven, with thousands of clouds and the sky around her.[26] The pain cave is not a secular metaphor but a deeply Christian one that taps into biblical stories and a medieval Western Christian church and Catholic worldview.[27] Marcia's pain cave illustrates the deep Christian frames that help CrossFitters make sense of the workout's pain during their activity and their relief after it is over.

When I asked Marcia where her pain cave imagery came from, she was confused. I had to walk her through the Christian elements before she informed me that they "probably" came from "being raised Christian." Her pain cave imagery seemed to stem from generic Christian themes—like hell being hot—rather than specific references to a Catholic literature of pilgrimage through doors (Dante), which was not part of her childhood or current faith. When I asked her if she was religious, she was quick to say, "Not anymore." She told me she learned as a psychology major during college that religion was a "comfort thing," "comfort in knowing there's this figure out there watching down on everyone and we all go heaven." She said she is now "okay with the uncomfortable" of not knowing what is going to happen, and she has since stopped praying to God for things. She no longer identifies as a Christian.

Although Marcia told me that she attended Bible camp once with a friend and church irregularly as a child, she spent much of her childhood at the CrossFit gym. She started going to CrossFit Kids (CK) when she was nine years old. Jeff and Mikki Martin created CK as a "turn-key" program, complete with lesson plans, magazine, and certification course, for affiliates wanting to cultivate "future generations of CrossFitters."[28] Marcia began attending this kids program dedicated to instilling CrossFit values and movements in children when she was in elementary school. Like many other kids, she went to CK while her mom attended a regular adult class. From ages fourteen to eighteen, Marcia coached CrossFit Kids alongside her mother. Marcia continued to do her own CrossFitting, spending hours at the gym when she was in her late teens and becoming "really good." When she turned twenty, she started teaching adult classes. At twenty-two, she currently lifts at a new CrossFit gym and hopes to begin coaching for it soon. Marcia was thus raised in a CrossFit gym, and it seems likely that her version of the pain cave comes more from hearing other CrossFitters talk about the pain cave than from Christian parables.

While Marcia used what I interpret as Christian themes in the description of her pain cave, this imagery comes from her somewhat-Christian-mainly-CrossFit upbringing. She was not even aware of her own use of what looks very much like Christian imagery until I brought it to her attention. Though she does not identify as a Christian any longer, it seems that she feels comfortable using these themes that resonate so strongly with Christianity because they seem like CrossFit themes. In other words, her understanding of pain and suffering was shaped by Christian imagery both in her Christian upbringing and in the Christian stories told at the CrossFit gym—environments that were suffused with culturally Christian concepts, though they seemed more "generic" and secular to her. The pain cave themes simply felt like *American CrossFit themes* to her, as she did not claim a Christian faith.

In the United States, the religious tradition used to understand pain as meaningful is the wake of Christianity, afterlives of church-based rhetoric. It is of course not necessary to be Christian to feel pain as meaningful, nor is it the case that all Christians feel a deeper meaning in their pain. Rather, when pain has deeper meaning, as it does in CrossFit, a "ready-to-use" interpretive framework in the United States is a culturally Christian salvation one. It is ready to use because it is a pervasive underlying code of meaning in the US that has been repackaged as "American" in the wake of Christianity.

The American Redemptive Self

Redemption and salvation stories are important for many Americans, including white Americans. A white American psychologist named Dan McAdams was trying to make sense of self-actualizing persons—those who have reached their full potential—who found themselves telling their personal stories in a narrative redemptive arc. Their redemption stories' narrative arc followed Rachel's: was lost, was challenged, found something that was lifesaving, and committed to the work of it. McAdams thought that these were universal life experiences and that humans everywhere used this narrative arc to understand their lives. It is common practice for psychology to understand cultural stories as universal human stories. McAdams was confronted with the reality that this is not actually the case while giving a talk in Europe. He shared his thesis that all humans go through this arc of redemption as they mature. A woman from the audience challenged his assertion that these were universal human stories. She said to him, "Professor McAdams, this is very interesting, but these life stories you describe, they seem so, well, *American*."[29] McAdams was caught off guard. He was using Erik Erikson's theory of human development (which is based on a white, male, middle-class American developmental trajectory), which argues that those who reach the generative stage of human development experience themselves and tell their personal story using themes and trajectories of suffering, redemption, and personal destiny. This Dutch woman reminded him that this was not a generic human story. It was a cultural story, an American story. McAdams reflects that because of this woman's comment, he went on to write *The Redemptive Self*, a book on the ways *Americans* (not all humans but Americans of all backgrounds) organize their life stories around themes of suffering, redemption, and personal destiny.

The American stories of suffering, redemption, and personal destiny that make up what McAdams calls the "American self" have an ancestor.[30] They did not emerge out of thin air and become "American." Rather, they use a Christian template of sin and salvation. W. Clark Gilpin argues that "personal and societal transformation in American culture" is based on the "Christian template of sin and salvation." The paired ideas of sin and salvation imply a "narrative of human transformation, a redemptive process that recovers human life from erroneous ways and reorients it toward an ultimate goal or a transcendent power through which life is fulfilled."[31]

This sin and salvation narrative can trace its roots to the foundation of American society, where a Protestant work ethic and settler Christian colonialism shaped the desire to fulfill a life's mission, to live a purposeful life. Like McAdams, other early American scholars, such as the psychologist William James and the philosopher Josiah Royce, thought the framework of sin and salvation to be part of the "human condition." Like McAdams, they argued that there is a "central aim" or purpose to each human life and that if this is not found, the life is "a failure." "To be saved is not simply to be brought to safety but to be set on a path, to embark on a journey, to reorder everyday life by means of regular, frequently rigorous spiritual disciplines."[32] But this is not a universal human condition. It is an "American condition" organized on white, Protestant values, as these are the most dominant in the United States.[33] To be "American" is to understand salvation not as an experience of safety but as a rigorous, disciplinary reordering of everyday life—much like Rachel's reordered life.

Part of the reason psychologists like James and McAdams keep framing these stories as universal rather than cultural is that the nature of the discipline of psychology is to look for universal human experiences. (In fact, the field of anthropology—which examines the ways people live and make meaning throughout the world—was established to argue against psychology's universalist frameworks.)[34] But that is almost impossible when the very discipline of searching for human universals is founded and organized in a particular historical and cultural location. It is because of this American historical and cultural location that these "human stories," which are really "American stories," are also deeply "Christian stories." The "Christian" part became "universal" and distinctly "American," I would argue, because psychology was founded to secularize theories of a universal Christian inner life.

Early American psychologists, like William James, John Dewey, and G. Stanley Hall, were trying to secularize American psychology. They sought to understand and examine the "self," not the "soul." However, their backgrounds are distinctly Protestant, with many of them sons of pastors or themselves former ministers. Their psychology, I argue, while seemingly secular, is infused with cultural Christianity. Because how can it not be? American psychology was founded by Christian men in a Christian context.[35] The "scientific" questions of American psychology are answered using Christian theology and thought.[36] This circumstance is revealed by McAdams even a century after the founding of American psychology, when he argues that a universal human self is organized around redemption as a means of self-actualization. Even though he revisits this claim and argues that this self is an American one rather than a universal one, he still makes the claim that redemption stories can be secular.

McAdams claims that redemptive stories can be secular by arguing that such stories fill various popular culture spaces, such as in *People* magazine. Cultural Christianity allows an American psychologist like McAdams to believe that redemptive stories are universal rather than cultural/American, and secular rather than Christian, because Christianity is cultural, and it profoundly shapes American society even when it is not explicitly intending to be "religious." As we have seen, Christian frameworks are sitting in the room with us already, even for people who do not identify as Christian or in spaces that seem secular—like psychology, like the gym.[37]

Community Suffering: The CrossFit Gym

As we saw earlier in Rachel's testimonial and Marcia's pain cave, cultural Christian narrative elements are infused in the practice of CrossFit. The salvation narrative and pain cave imagery can be understood within both a Christian and an American narrative framework. What is also clear in Rachel's testimonial is that her suffering and salvation are not experienced alone. There is a community that is organized around misery, pushing through that misery and finding success: salvation. This is part of the foundation of the CrossFit community. But it also indexes a cultural Christian community.

The chronic, sacred pain discussed earlier is part of what the religious scholar Judith Perkins describes as the Christian suffering self. There is significance and meaning in pain and suffering in Christianity, in the creation of a "suffering self" *and* a community of sufferers. Bodily pain and suffering, Perkins writes, "provided Christians with their community identity." Perkins also argues that this suffering self became an institutional tenet of the early Christian church: "Early Christian narrative representation has shown that it functioned to construct Christians as a community of suffers."[38] In other words, Christianity and a Christian collective identity are based on collective suffering and redemption. Glucklich supports this claim, writing that Christianity "is identified as a community through shared pain, at the center of which stands the sacrifice of Jesus."³⁹ This collective identity is partially organized through narrative, on the one hand, and the lived experience of pain and suffering, on the other.

Pain and transformation through suffering also provide CrossFitters with their community identity. CrossFit is predicated on suffering—the pain of workouts and the community that suffers the workouts together—and healing: CrossFit heals people from their previously sinful lives, and their bodies are now fit thanks to the healing power of CrossFit. The meaning that CrossFit gives to pain is a deep one, a "sacred" one. It is through the pain of the workout that one comes to understand what one is capable of. Without pushing one's limits—as Rachel's testimonial and Marcia's Christian-themed pain cave illustrate—one cannot be saved. Without pushing limits, one would not have a CrossFit workout. And a CrossFit workout is done with others, as a class, in a community.

* * *

The speakers are screaming Bieber's "Despacito" as the barbells clang on the floor, the whip of the jump rope swirls, and people grunt through burpees. I watch four men lie on the ground, arms splayed out like Christ on the cross, as ten people—seven women and three men—continue through the workout. I can feel the reverberations of the barbells through the floor as I stretch and watch. The WOD is a partner one, written like this:

> In teams of 2 with one partner working at a time, complete the following for time:
> 200 Double-Unders
> 100 Burpees
> 50 Deadlifts 185/125
> 100 Double-Unders
> 50 Burpees
> 25 Deadlifts

This means that people pair up and complete two hundred double-unders (a jump-rope skill in which with each jump, the rope goes twice under the feet), then one hundred burpees, then fifty deadlifts (men lifting 185 pounds, women 125 pounds), then back to the jump rope, more burpees, and then finally deadlifts to finish. Partners can separate the work in any way that makes sense. For example, one person can do all of the double-unders, and the other can do the deadlifts; or, as more commonly happens to allow each person to practice various skills, the first person does as many double-unders as they can, and then the next person does the same, switching back and forth in each exercise. The pair records their time. The work does not have to be split evenly (someone can do more than the other). But the goal is to move as fast as possible, which requires understanding each other's skills (e.g., Is one of you stronger in the deadlift, better at the jump-rope skill?).

The two men's pairs have finished, while the other groups (one mixed-gender group has two barbells for the different deadlift weights) slog on. Everyone is sweaty, red-faced, or hunched over with fatigue. The partner not working has her hands on her hips, while the other jumps or lifts. Over the next couple of minutes, more pairs finish, sprawling on the ground.

"Come on, Sarah. Let's go, Kristi," Jack cheers from the floor.

"Let's goooooo!" Travis yells from next to me as we wait for our class to begin when the current one ends.

"Don't forget to brace, Frank," Coach Peter tells a deadlifter. "Nice work, Lisa!" Coach high-fives a red-faced, super-sweaty Lisa, who is collapsed on the floor in her female CrossFit uniform of barely there shorts and sports bra only.

People grunt extra loudly on the final deadlift. Finally, Justin Bieber is turned down, and Coach turns to fourteen CrossFitters and says, "Well done, five o'clock! Now write your times on the whiteboard and put your stuff away for the next class. Cash-out is a walk around the block. Be sure to drink lots of water."

The first finished pairs begin putting barbells and plates away, high-fiving people as they do. The last finishers continue to lie on the ground. Kristi has her hand over her eyes to keep the lights out of her pounding head. Frank's arms are splayed out to his sides, and he stares ahead trying to catch his breath.

The next couple of minutes are a transition time, as the 5 p.m. class finishes and those who are here for the 6 p.m. class enter one of the two phonebooth-sized changing rooms in their work clothes and emerge in spandex outfits, muscles on display: Clark Kent to Superman. The finishing CrossFitters catch their breath. The waiting ones lace up their shoes. People commingle, sharing tales of pain and strategy: "My legs are still sore from yesterday's squats" or "The double-unders destroy your shoulders for the burpees so try and break those up" or "I won't be able to move my arms tomorrow." Those who are ending the workout walk around the block together, groaning, grumbling, and sharing. The new class members seek out a partner for the pending workout.

The gym smells like sweat. Outlines of sweaty bodies, known as "sweat angels," are evident on the rubber-matted floor as people collapsed postworkout. Pools of sweat reveal double-under or deadlift stations. We "six o'clockers" try to find dry or the least gross areas as Coach Peter calls us to circle and warm up. It is our turn. As the "five o'clock" CrossFitters finish up, they shout "good luck" to us. When we finish, the "seven o'clock" class will greet us with "well dones" and high fives.

The next day, I can barely move my arms. Everyday tasks—cooking, dressing, brushing my teeth—all hurt. No matter, I still show up at the gym the next day and the next, as do the other six o'clock regulars. We are ready for the next workout and the pain and suffering it delivers. A classic CrossFit adage on a gym wall sign—"It never gets easier; you just get better"—reminds us that the lingering pain never goes away, but if we keep coming to CrossFit, we will get faster, stronger, more physically and mentally able to endure it.

The pain of CrossFit workouts is notorious, and the lore can scare people off: A *New York Times* article titled "Getting Fit, Even If It Kills You" is a good example.[40] The article is about the connection between CrossFit and rhabdomyolysis, commonly called "rhabdo" in CrossFit, a condition caused by muscle fiber breakdown that is too much for the kidneys to handle, so the excess poisons the blood. People must seek emergency medical treatment for this condition; a friend of mine had to be hospitalized for four days for rhabdo from a CrossFit WOD in 2023. While rhabdomyolysis is not very common, people are supposed to push themselves during CrossFit workouts. As noted earlier, CrossFit's unofficial mascot is a clown named either "Pukey" or "Uncle Rhabdo," depending on the context.[41] He is "Pukey" when he is depicted as a puking clown with stars swirling around his head, sweaty, dazed, and physically sick from the workout. He is "Uncle Rhabdo" when he is depicted as a clown standing in a pool of blood and tethered to a dialysis machine to clear his blood and save his kidneys. These images are muraled on the CrossFit gym wall or emblazoned on T-shirts.[42]

Even if you do not puke or get rhabdo, CrossFit workouts, like the one described earlier, are designed to be painful in the moment and in the days to come. Some people vomit to expel toxins in the form of excessive lactic acid buildup in the blood. Lactic acid builds up during exercise and can make muscles sore in the moment, known as "acute muscle soreness." Or sometimes the pain begins hours or days later and is known as "delayed-onset muscle soreness" (DOMS). DOMS occurs as the body repairs exercised-induced torn muscle fibers. A common DOMS effect is that muscles are too sore to move or touch. Other lingering problems can be exercise-induced pulmonary edema, in which the lungs cannot keep up with the heart and begin to take on fluid. The body coughs to reflexively expel this fluid. In CrossFit, it is known as "Fran Lung" or "Fran Cough" because it is associated with a particular workout named Fran.[43] Fran Lung, exercise-induced coughing, can last for days.

Whether it is acute or delayed muscle soreness, puking, or coughing, CrossFit is known for its destruction of the body and for the pain this causes. This is part of what Rachel meant when she said she had to be "convinced" to try CrossFit and why she felt she had to be "super up front" about her "preconceived notions" and how CrossFit was a "fad that gets people hurt." During a workout of burpees, Rachel questions if she is "really cut out for this." This is why the workout can feel like "hell," conjuring images of a biblical belly of a beast or Dante's *Inferno*.

It is also why pushing through the pain and finishing can feel like heaven—and why Rachel finds herself committing, because she is pushed to her limits, past them even, as in the nutrition challenge. Earlier we saw Lisa, Sarah, Kristi, and Frank suffering in and after a CrossFit workout. The pain and misery they push through are necessary, important, meaningful. One should not quit because of the pain and misery but rather experience them as building community and meaning for those "who push themselves so hard. "I see pushing my body to the point where the muscles destroy themselves as a huge benefit of CrossFit," a former Army Ranger who was hospitalized with rhabdomyolysis told Cooperman of the *New York Times*.[44] It is the pain—not its absence—that indexes the sacred realm.

Furthermore, CrossFit pain and salvation occur in a community context; it is shared suffering. In this workout, the pain of the workout is directly shared between partners, one suffering and then the other when the pain of the first is too great. This elicits a bonding in the shared suffering, as during the switching, one never is fully without pain when the other stops and needs respite. Nonetheless, through partnerships, one cultivates a sense of shared pain in the pursuit of a completed workout. In CrossFit classes more generally, in WODs that are not partner workouts, the group of CrossFitters shares in pain and salvation together during a workout, as well as with the classes before and after them. There is a bearing witness to others' pain and the experience of one's own within a group context that builds a sense of community suffering, pain, and collective salvation. Moreover, the class environment enables people to push themselves beyond what they might normally do on their own. People do not want to let their partners down, be the slowest time on the whiteboard, or let down the people cheering for them. Yes, one can get rhabdo or puke when one works out alone, but it is less likely. The only people I have known to get rhabdo did so in a class setting, not wanting to push less hard in front of others. The group class and partner workouts normalize CrossFit's pain and suffering, giving them redemptive meaning.

Conclusion

Rachel did not want to do CrossFit; she had heard all the negative things. But her proselytizing coworker convinced her, and she gave it a try. Soon, she found herself transformed, saved by the shared pain of the workouts and camaraderie forged in that pain. Her story reads like an Augustinian confession, complete with being lost, finding Jesus/Christianity/CrossFit, and being transformed and saved. We also heard Marcia tell us about her pain in a CrossFit workout: her story of the (hell) cave and her subsequent appearance on the mountain peak. Her story resonates deeply with various versions of Christian stories of hell and salvation, even though she probably learned them more at the CrossFit gym than at Sunday school. As we saw in the description of the painful workout, it is the lived experience of the pain that grounds the salvation stories. Salvation is found in the pain, in the suffering but not failing, in the community of fellow sufferers committed to being better versions of themselves. This salvation is part of the community of CrossFit, a community of people organized around certain values and practices, including, importantly, finding self-transformative meaning in shared pain and suffering.

CrossFit self-transformation comes during the workouts but also in the hours outside the gym. You will find yourself thinking about CrossFit and the workouts outside the gym if the double-unders prevent you from typing at your computer without pain or if you cough for days. This is how CrossFit becomes what Madeline Ulrich describes as "a huge part of your life. Somehow everything goes back to CrossFit when you do CrossFit."[45] It is hard to compartmentalize and leave CrossFit pain in the gym when that pain takes over your life. The pain when typing is a constant reminder that you pushed yourself hard at the gym, that you will do so again tomorrow, that you should eat "better" and drink more water to help with the recovery and to prepare for the next trauma from tomorrow's surprise workout. The pain is also triumphant; it continuously interrupts your otherwise non-CrossFit life to remind you that you did this really hard thing, and you should be proud of that achievement. It also reminds you that you could do it again, or something more challenging, something heroic. Perhaps, in classic CrossFit's framework of preparing for the unknown, you would have the fortitude and strength to escape your white-collar office building, with a coworker slung over your shoulder, in the event of an earthquake, a bombing, or the end times. This salvation finds purchase in the brand of CrossFit, sold by a modern-day oracle.

3

CrossFit Capitalism

Oracles and Garages

In 2013, Greg Glassman addressed an audience at the State Policy Network, a group interested in fostering entrepreneurial and community endeavors. Glassman stands at a lectern. He is wearing a button-up shirt, and his hair is slicked back (remarkably different attire from the *60 Minutes* interview we have seen him in). He is speaking about his founding of CrossFit and the company's subsequent growth. The video of the speech is posted on the CrossFit webpage for the company's magazine, the *CrossFit Journal*, and thirty-five comments praise it.

In the video, Glassman talks about being kicked out of all the commercial gyms in his town, being allowed space in a client's jiujitsu gym, and after about a year of that, opening his own gym and the first-ever CrossFit box. It was in an industrial space with a giant rolled-up garage door, on the edge of the city of Santa Cruz. As he discusses the prototype of most CrossFit gyms to come, he describes his fears about being a good businessman, as he followed a checklist of pros and cons: "What I was doing, my checklist was really about, 'Will this work financially?' 'Is this a good business decision?' And the mind-set was that business is about making money. If you can't pay the rent, you won't be in business. But then it hit me in just a blinding flash that, wait a minute, I'm not trying to make money. Money's what happens when you do something right."[1]

A little bit later in the speech, Glassman talks about the relationship he has with "an outfit called Rogue." CrossFit helped make it possible for Rogue to be a successful business also: "Let me give you one for instance. There's an outfit called Rogue. They're in Columbus, Ohio. They make CrossFit gear; they make equipment for CrossFitters. They'll probably do $60 million this year. Now, I could help myself to some of that by requiring that affiliates use CrossFit-branded gear, and then Rogue would have a real problem. I don't want to own Rogue. I don't want to step outside of our core competency. *I don't want to lose the moral authority.* I'm not trying to make money. I'm trying to grow a community." He concludes the speech with, "Money is essential to run a business, but it's not *why* you run a business, and it's not what makes a business grow. Businesses grow on dreams. Trying to make money is no way to run a business."[2] In the comments, people praise Glassman's speech:

"We are incredibly lucky to have you as our leader."[3]
"Another example of why CrossFit is the best thing in the world."[4]
"This is everything I have ever dreamed of. To be part of this community is beyond words. Thank you, Greg Glassman, for creating this for the world. You have started a legacy of a positive, co-creative community that will raise consciousness of everything everywhere."[5]
"Thanks must be given to Coach for his ingenuity, for his integrity, and for never selling out to those who are interested in making him rich. I bet he sleeps very well each night knowing that He [sic] is the wealthiest man in the world. His gift to us is simple: Go out and excel at your craft, enjoy the coaching, enjoy the teaching enjoy each person you come in contact with, live in the moment and create change in those that come in contact with you. So simple and so altruistic that it boggles the mind that it hadn't been created. I am so thankful that I am able to come to my gym and turn the lights on and just dream of making a change in my community's lives. Thank you, Coach Glassman. CrossFit Northland in Kansas City."[6]
"The world has hope with people like Coach in it."[7]
"Guru is the WORD I now use for coach G. Thanks, you give me hope in humanity NAMASTE!"[8]

By 2017, CrossFit was the seventh-largest and fastest-growing corporate chain in the world, alongside Subway (#1), McDonald's (#2), and Pizza Hut (#6). At that time, it was the largest fitness chain in the world, with fifteen thousand locations in 162 countries.[9] Despite Glassman's mantra that businesses grow on dreams and that he was leaving money on the table, CrossFit was making money hand over fist.

After Glassman's blinding flash of insight, his "aha!" moment if you will, in which he realized that it was not about money but about pursuing excellence and letting the money follow, he seemed to do both: make a lot of money and establish a community and fitness method that was excellent. Digging through the *CrossFit Journal*, I came across another video from 2012, before he gave the formal lecture to the State Policy Network and before his was the largest fitness chain in the world. In this video, he is clearer about his commitment to "leaving money on the table":

> Let me tell you what is left on the table. It's the seed capital for the affiliates to grow their businesses. It's the opportunity for friends like Rogue and Beyond the Whiteboard to do a better job of things, to commit to products and services that we don't have the resources to provide. It's a college savings plan for the affiliates and their trainers, for their kids. We control a very, very small percent of the CrossFit financial ecosystem, and that's by design. That's by design. If we insert ourselves in this, if we start to see the points of presence, see our affiliates as economic opportunity for rent extraction, we have to alter our relationship with them. And we abandoned this *covenant*, this charter that is *sacred* to all of us, and we kill the very thing that is making this *revolution* possible.[10]

Here, we see terms like "sacred," "covenant," and "revolution" being used as the reasons for leaving money on the table. The relationship that CrossFit HQ has with the affiliates or local gym owners and other CrossFit-born businesses (Rogue, Beyond the Whiteboard) is, according to Glassman, not about money. It is about keeping to a sacred contract that the company made as part of its fitness revolution. Greg Glassman and the business of CrossFit grew on moral authority to pursue what he calls "excellence" over money. Money would follow the excellence, and during the first two decades of the twenty-first century, CrossFit, affiliate owners, and companies like Rogue would flourish. They would find "buy in" to a business model that focuses on dreams, excellence, and community over bottom-line profits. This, Glassman argued, was in direct contrast to venture capitalists who told him he left too much money on the table by limiting his cut of the pie. Unlike venture capitalists, small business owners like those we see in the comments praise Glassman for making it possible for them to live their dreams, change their communities, raise consciousnesses, and enhance people's lives. The final comment quoted earlier praises Glassman for giving him hope in humanity, identifying him as a "guru."

What does it mean that a company is both one of the fastest growing and largest corporate chains and that it sees itself as having moral authority by leaving money on the table, using a sacred covenant with its affiliates, and mobilizing a revolution? What does it mean that those who follow this fitness program think of the founder and CEO as a guru who provides hope to the world? It is not hard to get a sense that CrossFit is a beloved "brand," that the creator is a beloved leader or even "guru," and that this economic strategy—of leaving money on the table—is not a common one in neoliberal America. So, what kind of economic strategy is it? What kind of capitalism lends itself to CrossFit being such a beloved *branded* community with a guru-like leader?

It is useful to examine the different forms of capitalism that allowed CrossFit to become as popular as it has. At the end of the twentieth century and beginning of the twenty-first, the internet was taking off, Oprah could change markets with pithy statements or by endorsing books, and the United States was attacked on September 11, 2001.

CrossFit began as a brick-and-mortar, garage-type gym in Santa Cruz, based on the roguish and savant-like (revolutionary?) training behavior turned methodology of its creator, Greg Glassman. This training methodology focused on being constantly varied, functional, and intense. Glassman also posted his daily workouts (WODs) on the internet at the CrossFit website. Anyone could visit the site, get free training advice in the form of a workout, and post about it, thereby building the foundation of CrossFit's beloved community.

This community would grow. Many of the first members of the community were people in the military or police, as the methodology was linked to preparation for fighting terrorism. People wanted to build their own CrossFit gyms, akin to martial arts studios rather than franchises, and an affiliate system was forged. The affiliate system was antifranchise; it required a small annual fee ($1,000–$3,000) and "left money on the table." This approach allowed people with less financial capital to open a CrossFit gym and to use their profits to invest in their communities, not pay rent to CrossFit. It allowed for dreams to flourish, rather than simply venture capitalists' profits, giving Glassman his moral authority, as his model encouraged America's small business ideology. Glassman's entrepreneurial spirit, however, builds on other forms of US capitalism, particularly what I call *oracle capitalism*, akin to Oprah with her ability to amass followers with self-transformative endeavors, and what I call *garage capitalism*, as he was another "white male college dropout in a garage in California," much like Apple's and Disney's founders. The link with the military did not begin with CrossFit; physical fitness in the US has always been linked to the US military. Yet CrossFit's constantly varied functional fitness at high intensity to prepare one for unknown physical fitness tests fit right into the country's fears and anxieties in a post-9/11 world, where everyday Americans needed an oracle in a garage to help them realize their capitalist and fitness dreams.

Oracle Capitalism

In the early to mid-1990s, daytime television consisted of various talk shows. According to scholars, these talk shows were identified as "trash-talk TV." Oprah, who had been a leader in the genre, was seeing her ratings decline and decided to "cease focusing on dysfunction and start emphasizing positive topics."[11] By the end of the decade, Oprah and her show eclipsed all other shows, and she became a "prophet" and "one of the most trusted brand names" in the US.[12] She transformed herself and her talk show into a media empire that included a website, a book club, a magazine, a radio show, personal growth tours, a Facebook page, a YouTube channel, and a cable TV station. Oprah Winfrey became simply "Oprah," and her recommendations had what was identified as "the Oprah effect," which could alter stock markets.[13] Her focus on "positive topics" came to be known as "Change Your Life Television," in which she served as an oracle for the millions of (mostly) white women who tuned in. Oprah transformed herself from talk-show host to media mogul, celebrity, and icon spreading good news.

According to the religious studies scholar Kathryn Lofton, what matters for understanding Oprah, and, I would argue, others who follow in similar footsteps, "is that this explicitly missionary maneuver to help people was her empire's ascent."[14] Oprah tapped into what the psychologist Steven Starker argues is the eternal optimism of the American spirit and consumer, as evinced in the form of self-help.[15] Oprah epitomized the genre of self-help, which has roots as deep in American Christianity as it does in the field of psychology, and she soon became an oracle.

The notion of an oracle is key here. An oracle is often understood as a woman with divine wisdom. The most well-known, perhaps, was the Oracle at Delphi, Greece, whose inscription was "Know Thyself." The term "oracle" has Latin origins meaning "to speak," but oracles can be found across cultures and histories. What an oracle does is provide wisdom, wise counsel, or even prophetic insights about how best to live. Often, oracles have religious roots, and their speech acts are divinations. In the United States, Starker argues, the oracle, with its wise counsel on how best to live, is not located in a remote village in the mountains of Greece but can be found in the literature of American Christianity and popular psychology. Starker argues that in the United States, the most common oracle is "at the supermarket," in the form of self-help books. He published his book long before the height of the talk-show era of Oprah or the proliferation of psychology-speak on Instagram and TikTok. But his essential argument is still pertinent. The search for pithy answers to life's problems and questions is not an American phenomenon, but finding them in a mass-produced way through icons of good news is.

Starker identified thirty-seven hundred books with the title "how to" between 1983 and 1984, but these books were just the tip of the self-help-oracle-at-the-supermarket iceberg. They were, in fact, part of a long tradition of good-news preachers and mind-cure advocates. Self-help literature has been a wildly popular genre in the United States, reflecting popular understandings of the "self" that needed help and the historical and cultural context that supported the literature. Starker traces the beginning back to Cotton Mather and his Puritan-inspired essays "to do good" (1710) and Benjamin Franklin and his book *The Way to Wealth* (1757).[16] But he focuses on the end of the nineteenth and turn of the twentieth centuries and the Puritan publications that proposed that people follow mainstream Protestant ethics, including those found in the Brooklyn clergyman Wilbur F. Crafts's *Successful Men* (1883).[17]

In the early 1900s, the New Thought movement took shape, providing a "new philosophy" through less fundamental religious frameworks. New Thought, an American Protestant religious movement beginning in the late 1800s that focused on mind-over-matter thinking and that explicitly linked corporeality with spirituality, argued that salvation was found through health, diet, fasting, sexual restraint, and fitness regimens. For example, following the 1929 Wall Street Crash, the self-help literature used New Thought theology to promote the cultivation of financial wealth, including in Napoleon Hill's *Think and Grow Rich* (1937) and Dale Carnegie's *How to Win Friends and Influence People* (1937). Both books were published in Simon and Schuster's paperback "Pocket Books," which revolutionized the publishing industry.

Both volumes also reflected the growing influence of "psychology" outside of the academy beginning in the 1930s. In 1952, Norman Vincent Peale's *The Power of Positive Thinking* linked New Thought theology with the powerful voice of a mainstream clergyman who wrote in positive psychology-speak. The 1960s self-help books reflected changes in social mores and included works that moved past official Christian theology and popularized psychological theory, such as Abraham Maslow's development theory and self-actualization and Carl Rogers's work on "personality." The 1980s included more diet, exercise, and financial divinations through the oracles at the supermarket. It was in the 1980s that the "calorie" became known as a unit of understanding food and "nutrition" became an academic subject, both popularized by the self-help literature and the use of talk-show television. Starker's book was published in 1989, and thus the 1980s is the last decade he examines.

What is clear is that many of the popular books from earlier decades remain relevant today, as do many of their topics of inquiry. *The Power of Positive Thinking* is still wildly popular, and three *Shark Tank* judges swear by Hill's *Think and Grow Rich* as *the* self-help book on wealth-building.[18] While the authors of those books are no longer with us, their use of New Thought theology as oracle wisdom remains.

Thus, Oprah did not emerge out of nowhere. Her oracle empire, built on positive thinking and missionary zeal, is the result of a long historical and cultural tradition of linking American Christian thought, specifically New Thought theology and mainline Protestantism, with popular media, without being overt about its Christian roots.[19] While Oprah professes to be Christian and to have honed her public speaking skills in the pulpit, many people see her as more of a "New Age" guru who gives a platform to "Higher Beings" and "Secrets" rather than to Jesus Christ. While this critique might be valid, her roots are Christian, and her ability to reach the masses in her oracle form is precisely because of the afterlives of Christian self-help/salvation narratives disguised as pop psychology at the supermarket. Cultural Christianity is sitting in the supermarket already, an underlying code shaping self-help books.

What Oprah has done beyond that of the generic oracle at the supermarket is to link her wisdom to her person and transform herself from Oprah Winfrey the woman to Oprah the brand. Unlike a bookshelf of various self-help books from a variety of oracles, Oprah's wise counsel came to dominate, and her choice of anything—communicated via her talk show, satellite radio station, book club, magazine, brick-and-mortar store, or television channel—directed consumers' consumption choices. Product placement in self-help narratives linked self-help habits and practices with products. Oprah told (mostly white, mostly female) Americans to keep a gratitude journal—and what kind of journal to buy. Her product placement was not just crass; each item was linked to her good news and the ways to put that good news to work. For example, in her penchant for gift-giving, Oprah learned that a New York City police officer who was at Ground Zero on 9/11 kept a gratitude journal; Oprah gave this police officer a new journal, from Oprah's favorite line of journals, and a beautiful Rebecca Moss pen to use in her gratitude writing.[20] This gesture linked a self-transformation habit (gratitude journaling) with a product (favorite journal and pen) with American nationalism (a police officer from Ground Zero) in one gift-giving event. This did not happen only once. This kind of thing was Oprah's brand: an oracle dispensing self-help wisdom by recommending practice and product, both altruistic gifts to her fans.

What does this have to do with CrossFit or Greg Glassman? In an episode of *The Oprah Winfrey Show*, Oprah is talking with Michael Beckwith, a teacher of *The Secret* (a contemporary New Thought theology book), and she says, "Nobody, including myself and Bill Gates (know him personally), was trying to make money.... You have to follow what is the thing that gives you your juice."[21] Oprah attests that she was not trying to make money. She just followed her dreams to help people, and her desire for excellence and to keep things positive, and voilà, there she was, an oracle to the masses of white American women, her "juice" shaping the political economics of American society. It is this following of dreams or juice that leads Oprah to become less profit-hungry businesswoman and more prophet-like giver of consumptive advice that makes people like her oracles. Glassman is similar. He maintains that he did not endeavor to make money; money is what happens when you do the right thing. It is very Protestant ethic, very Prosperity Gospel, or the American Christian belief that God wants believers to prosper in health and wealth.[22] And doing the right thing confers moral authority to those who are not profit-driven and rent-extracting.

Greg Glassman, the creator, cofounder, and voice of CrossFit, took a similar approach as Oprah. Because of his decisions to get his personal training clients off the ellipticals, leg-extension machines, and carbs, he became an outlier in mainstream physical fitness. He established a new training method that was constantly varied, using functional movements performed at high intensity. He called this "CrossFit"—less precise than "Change Your Life Television," but the results were similar. His early days were in a friend's jiujitsu studio and then a small garage gym that he outgrew in five months. He went online with CrossFit.com, next door in Santa Cruz to a bigger space, and across the country through newly established affiliates. He became the oracle of physical fitness, providing the correct kinds of movements and preaching their practice at high intensity. Glassman wrote prolifically in the *CrossFit Journal*, a monthly newsletter that one could receive in the mail or find online. He used print and online media to get his sage wisdom out to the masses, and many heard his call. However, it was the coaching courses and affiliate system that exponentially transformed the economics of CrossFit. It is this dedication to the local that enables Glassman to maintain his moral authority.

The affiliate system is different from a franchise; it requires a yearly fee for the use of the name "CrossFit." That is it. Neither CrossFit nor Glassman gives advice on any other business-related topics. In fact, he argues, he gives his training regimen out for free on the internet, he writes about various business-related things (such as how to outfit a garage gym) in his journal, and he gives talks around the country and then posts them on his website. None of this comes at a financial cost to the general CrossFit enthusiast. What does cost is the training course to become a CrossFit coach, and this is required to open a CrossFit gym.

Unlike Oprah, Glassman was also a teacher, and his followers included fans as well as students/disciples. He decided that affiliates needed to have certified CrossFit coaches and that he would train them.

To become an affiliate, one needed to apply. Included in the application was a proposed name of the gym, evidence you had taken a CrossFit Level 1 training course, and an essay about how CrossFit had changed your life and how you would change your community, akin to the public testimonials discussed earlier. Glassman essentially created CrossFit disciples, each opening their own gym.

The CrossFit gym as an affiliate is reminiscent of the American congregationalist church. Each church has a pastor who is beholden to members of the congregation, those who live in the community. Unlike hierarchical Christian systems in which Catholic priests or Episcopalian bishops are placed somewhere by church leaders (or the church's polity), congregationalist churches are led by congregations and pastors.[23] Pastors are hired by the democratic church, the entire congregation having a say in who is pastor and in other church matters. CrossFit affiliates are led by gym owners or head coaches who have been granted an affiliate name and coaching ability by CrossFit HQ, but they are successful based on being known, respected, and accepted by the local community, culturally Christian congregationalist style.

In addition, CrossFit does not require local affiliates to pay Glassman any of the money they make, besides the annual affiliation fee to use the name "CrossFit." The money that gym owners make goes into their pockets, into a "college savings plan" for their kids or trainers, into new equipment that they want or like, perhaps one built by a local welder rather than one designated by CrossFit. This is Glassman's sacred covenant with gym owners: I will not tell you what to do or demand anything from you except the yearly fee and reupping your certification every five years. This is how businesses grow—CrossFit HQ and local affiliates—through dreams and commitments to sacred covenants. It is this that Glassman argues is the fitness revolution.

The community of CrossFit is both local and global. One goes to one's local box, knows the owner, and is friends with members. Members pay a lot of money to show up to what is identified as "the best hour of their day" and sweat together. They do burpees together. They also then party together. This is the agony and the laughter that forges a strong community, a beloved community of people who follow the oracle of CrossFit, constantly varied functional movement at high intensity, and the vision of Glassman: non-rent-extracting, dream-following encouragement, physical fitness, small business ownership, and beloved community all wrapped into one. CrossFit as physical fitness, small business ownership, and beloved community is also global. Each of the fifteen thousand boxes dedicates itself to its local community.

Boxes around the world also provide a pilgrimage site, as they invite their fellow CrossFitters to drop in and break a sweat in the fellowship of CrossFit. To show that you have made this pilgrimage, the community has a souvenir, one that any CrossFitter anywhere in the world would recognize as one of their own: the CrossFit gym T-shirt. The scholar of religion Alexander Ornella argues in his work on CrossFit T-shirts that T-shirts "play an important role in expressing the workout mentality and mindset, values, gender roles (or their subversion), and in embodying, rendering visible, and knitting together the global CrossFit community."[24] This is not unique to CrossFit; T-shirts are part of sport fandom. But unlike identifying someone as just a fan, the local gym's CrossFit T-shirt, especially those bought during travel, operates as a sort of pilgrim badge along the lines of souvenirs that pilgrims purchase at local sacred sites to show they made the journey.[25] Across the world, the "badge" is the same: a T-shirt with the name of the gym, "CrossFit [Something]," and maybe an image of the local mascot. This T-shirt is immediately recognizable as a badge from a local CrossFit gym. Gyms might also be gifted a T-shirt from a person who drops in, representing their home gym, and these are often hung around the gyms. Like the crosses of Christianity, head scarves of Islam, or yarmulkes of Judaism, the CrossFit T-shirt, a sort of pilgrimage badge to another CrossFit site, is recognized as representing the local community where one practices and the global community of practitioners. It is a tangible expression of one's faith in and devotion to CrossFit and the CrossFit community.

The beloved community has its oracle, with the message of following one's dreams. It is shared by people all over the world, represented in their pilgrim badges of CrossFit T-shirts. The beloved community also has its leader, its guru, who carefully made use of the garage to create an identity and origin story that tapped into the American entrepreneurial trope of the garage as the birthplace of ingenuity and revolution.

Garage Capitalism

In addition to oracle capitalism, CrossFit also shares a common origin story with other successful American companies and brands. Eric Lemay writes, "CrossFit begins with a guy in his garage, tinkering around and inventing something revolutionary. Think Thomas Edison, think Steve Jobs and Bill Gates."[26] The guy in his garage in the 1990s is a classic Silicon Valley trope: all innovative things come from this location, a common origin story for elite American entrepreneurs, rogue white men who dropped out of the wider world to focus on their passion and, eventually, bring it to the marketplace. Natalia Petrzela writes in her book *Fit Nation* that the CrossFit brand hinged on being an "anti-gym."[27] CrossFit distinguished itself from other fitness brands in the competitive, extensive marketplace of fitness by rejecting mainstream fitness practices and capitalizing on its garage origins, the location of revolutionary figures.

The garage holds a particular position in American culture. Olivia Erlanger and Luis Ortega Govela argue that it is a lens through which to view much of dominant American mythology. They write,

> Frank Lloyd Wright invented the garage when he moved the automobile out of the stable and into a room of its own. Steve Jobs and Steve Wozniak (allegedly) started Apple Computer in a garage. Suburban men turned garages into man caves to escape from family life. Nirvana and No Doubt played their first cords as garage bands. What began as an architectural construct became a cultural construct. . . . The garage was an aboveground underground. . . .
>
> The garage is an institution built upon an infrastructure of images. The proto-garage, the stable, was depicted in nativity scenes as the birthplace of Christianity, and as it transformed into the attached garage it has since been painted as the Eden of Silicon Valley, Disney, and Nirvana. From Bill Gates to Gwen Stefani, new American heroes thirsty for neoliberal liquidity were sheltered in this space. In their process of *garagification* these characters also became an image that seemingly overthrows the established order.[28]

Created to hold the car and synonymous with the suburbanization of American society, the garage has come to dominate the façade of the house, illustrating the "impact this space had on the suburban nuclear family."[29] It is a normative space, another room in the single-family home of middle-class heteronormative white America. But this normative space was also unique, a "blank canvas" with its open space and bare floors. As such, it could hold the car, but it could also be used for other manly pursuits, a frontier-like space where men could resist the domesticity of the suburban household. Its vibe is one of potential and authenticity; one could find freedom in the garage and, with it, a glorification of the individual, an entrepreneurial spirit, or punk or teenage angst. The garage housed men tinkering away on their machines or creating new ones that would change the world.

The garage is central to the tech-industrial complex in Silicon Valley, where several corporate success stories have emerged: Hewlett-Packard, Disney, Google, Amazon, and Apple. While the venture capitalist soon found these men hiding away in the garage, the aura of punk or resistance remains in the garage ethos. The garage as a workspace within the domestic space allowed for an "entrepreneurial ethos of work disguised as leisure," a space almost designed for a "do-it-yourself attitude," where the amateur could evolve into a "disruptive" expert.[30]

With these stories of garage heroes came the *garage myth*, which is based on concepts of self-reliance and individualism, mobilized by men who needed a room of their own, a cave that indexed a return to primordialism. The "garage functioned as a conductor for new thinking, new subjectivities that would forge new identities and actions." The garage became "an incubator for the entrepreneurial subject emerging from the high pressure, success-oriented, individualist America. Once the garage was dwelled in, occupied, and appropriated by start-up culture, it began to recycle and fabricate memories and myths that have supported its iconography as the space of invention.... Tenants use it as a dream box for reinvention, for rebranding their selfhoods."[31]

For Glassman, the garage became the place where he could train his clients without being thrown out, where he could practice his new fitness method, and where he could realize his dream. It was in a garage—first in his parents' house and then in a gym he founded in Santa Cruz, in the industrial park with the rolled-up garage door—that Glassman's CrossFit was born. He did not know he was going to be as successful as he became when he emerged from the garage, but CrossFit's founding and ethos are examples of the garage myth. A man tinkering away on his blank canvas, allowing his primordial instincts to be harnessed into "constantly varied functional movement at high intensity." CrossFit did not just emerge from a garage, with all the mythos and ethos of the garage myth. It also encouraged others, the soon-to-be affiliates, to do the same: build your own business in your garage, following our example, and call it CrossFit.

The second-ever volume of the *CrossFit Journal* (September 2002) is titled "The Garage Gym." The issue includes "how to" create a "world-class strength and conditioning facility in your garage," a list of equipment suppliers and vendors, a list of equipment to buy, how to forge a garage gym on a budget, a guide for getting "kicked out of your [local, mainstream] gym in ten days or less!" and an image of a bully-breed dog face at the top left corner, with a caption of "mess you up."[32] The issue provides a solution to a local mainstream gym that is a twenty-thirty-minute commute, plays music "worse than annoying," where the staff are "worthless," where the "place is packed with selectorized equipment for which we [CrossFit] have no use," and which is predicated on the bodybuilding model of physique development rather than on serious sport or military training. The list of ways to get kicked out of your local gym includes playing AC/DC's "Thunderstruck," grunting, screaming, using chalk during heavy deadlifts, climbing support poles around the gym, and working out with your shirt off and, if this does not get a reaction, having your girlfriend or wife take hers off.[33] All of these things one can do in one's own garage; thus, if you get kicked out, do not worry. The solution is to build your own garage gym. Your garage, stuffed with "15 years of junk," is "begging to become a gym." Move the car to the driveway (cover it, if you must), build a storage shed in the backyard, and you are on your way to the gym of your dreams. "If cost is an objection you may consider reevaluating your priorities," because "we're waging this revolution in your home. That's the only place it can be won."[34]

One easily picks up on the contrarian tone of the issue. Glassman, like many garage entrepreneurs who seek to transform the world, is known for it. He had been kicked out of many mainstream gyms for his oppositional behavior to gym norms. He probably did everything on the list of how to get kicked out of the local gym and then some. With this contrarian tone and ideas framed as "revolutionary," CrossFit and Glassman will take on big-gym to save folks from poor metabolic health due to an inferior workout regimen based on body-building exercises. The revolution will not be televised. It will be in your garage. CrossFit revolution is firmly situated within this middle-class, nerdy-punk white guy toying away in his garage, who finds a solution to a current problem and then brings that solution to the people. I call this *garage capitalism*, and it is predicated on the following elements.

First, the garage is a solidly middle-class architectural element that is firmly embedded in suburbia. One cannot find solace or revolution in their garage if one is not lucky enough to have one. But the garage is not just a middle-class space, as it is not fully embedded into the suburban home. It is either attached to or next to the home; therefore, it is not completely part of the home. Its adjacent status and "blank canvas" openness allow for creative use.

Second, the garage holds the mystique of being an "aboveground underground," as it is a room or space on the *edge* of, but firmly attached to, suburban, domestic, heteronormative, middle-class space. One might be lucky enough to have a garage, but one might not really fit within the confines of the rigidly ordered domestic. Take Greg Glassman: his origin story is that his father was an engineer/rocket scientist for Hughes Aircraft who taught Glassman the need to quantify and measure everything, and his mother was a homemaker. Glassman was raised in a solidly middle-/upper-middle-class Christian household.[35] At the same time, Glassman was a small kid with a limp from childhood polio and a chip on his shoulder, a "college dropout" who had been fired from all the personal training jobs in mainstream gyms he had. He would do workouts with his friends in his garage, going so hard that he made himself and his friends puke. He was not a domesticated suburbanite. He was a rogue. For Glassman, the garage is both a suburban middle-class luxury and a space in which to forge a revolution, as it is for others in this genre.

Third, the garage is known in California as fertile ground for the tinkering of smart men who bring new ideas and inventions to the world. Erlanger and Govela write that the garage is part of a myth of self-reliance and individualism and of a version of the American hero; it is the birthplace of a cis-male-dominated modernist movement. It is a space "of initiation and transition, the sacred space where characters can fight against the context that surrounds them to construct themselves anew: a temple to the self."[36] In the second volume of the *CrossFit*

Journal, CrossFit demands that one transform one's garage into a gym, prioritizing one's health and physical fitness above consumption. Make the garage a temple to the self.

Fourth, the garage is mythologized. Yes, it is a physical place, but it is a culturally constructed place. If CrossFit was forged in a garage, then the affiliates themselves would create their own gyms to resemble that garage space. The "anti-gym" is the garage. And because Glassman created his first CrossFit workouts in his garage and then opened the first CrossFit in an industrial space, complete with a garage roll-up door, the ideal CrossFit gym would also resemble a garage, regardless of an affiliate's need to begin in one. A July 2005 *CrossFit Journal* article titled "Garage Gym II—The Revolution" revisits "the CrossFit garage-gym concept to report on the successes of what may be hundreds of CrossFit start-up gyms and the aspirations and motivations of the people behind them."[37] The garage gym started as one's individual garage makeover and quickly became the "start-up" gym style of choice for newly established formal CrossFit affiliates around the country and world, including in major world cities such as London and New York and at military outposts in "Puerto Rico, Baghdad, Afghanistan, and Qatar."[38]

The big-box or masculine gym was the initial enemy, but Curves was a close second. The garage-type location for a CrossFit gym was a small box; thus, the name "CrossFit box" stuck. The small box is not just a scaled-down version of the big box. Rather, it was the antithesis of the big box, where feelings of alienation and the realities of being kicked out of mainstream gyms germinate. Curves was a profoundly popular fitness brand in the early 2000s. It was a small boutique gym that promised an effective thirty-minute circuit-training program designed to tone muscles. More importantly, it was *for women*. CrossFit, on the other hand, was not boutique-like. It was in a garage, the location of the "man cave," the primordial refuge, a place "where, regardless of gender, the inhabitants learn the codes of masculinity."[39] CrossFit was a masculine answer to this women-only fitness craze. And in this box/garage, the CrossFit brand was built on the mythology of masculine alienation that is housed and cultivated in the garage. According to Glassman in his "The Garage Gym II,"

> The best of what CrossFit offers, effective programming and constructive community, it does so for free. The family of trainers and trainees

working under the CrossFit banner are motivated, to varying degrees, by duty to country, camaraderie, job description, athletic dream, self-improvement, and profit. . . . CrossFit is an Internet-based grassroots movement giving call to all who really care about fitness to get the car out of the garage . . . and try the Workout of the Day. We want to fuel a revolution in fitness. . . . We know this can be done in the little boxes and we've proven that the garage is as good an environment as any for forging elite fitness.[40]

Alongside these statements are twenty-one images of various CrossFit boxes/garage gyms, illustrating the mythology of CrossFit's birthplace and revolution. The garage became an ideal for CrossFit affiliates around the world to establish their own anti-gym. A mythology that one can believe in, Douglas Atkin writes in his book *The Culting of Brands*, "leads to a long term relationship between company and customers," as "the self-made entrepreneurs strive to create #believers out of their customers."[41] Merging garage mythology with believing customers, CrossFit, in the wake of Christianity, links the garage (stable) with the oracle, the birthplace of a revolutionary with a mission in his message.

Erlanger and Govela write, "The most interesting aspect of the garage is not that it has created revolution but ultimately that it is always attached to the traditional values of a suburban home; the radical inventions that happened within it still reinforced the patriarchal capitalism and gendered domesticity from which they emerged."[42] The CrossFit garage-gym was built on the mythology of the garage forged by entrepreneurs in California who found refuge from corporate America and the cult of domesticity and cultivated new punk identities and innovative items in this masculine space. The garage is for the entrepreneur, the angsty teenager rebelling against the world, the punk (band or gym bro) who wants to throw tires and scream loudly. CrossFit is for the masculine, the tough, the rogue.

Rogue Fitness

In January 2013, at the State Policy Network's twentieth annual meeting, discussed earlier, Greg Glassman told the audience about his business strategy, "Businesses grow on dreams, not money," and provided an example of how he supports the individual entrepreneurial spirit and dreams of other entities, besides CrossFit, such as "an outfit called Rogue."

If you go to Rogue's website and the "About Us" page, you will read a similar origin story to CrossFit, born in a garage because of the need to fill that garage with proper workout equipment. Like CrossFit, Rogue is currently a very successful business dedicated to the needs of serious athletes or garage gym enthusiasts. "Rogue Fitness is the leading manufacturer of strength and conditioning equipment, including barbells, power racks, sleds, and accessories. Founded in a garage in 2006, the company has grown to over 1400 team members globally. Rogue is the official equipment supplier of the CrossFit Games, USA Weightlifting, the Arnold Strongman Classic, and the World's Strongest Man competition. The company remains dedicated to serving the needs of serious athletes at every level, from the garage to the arena."[43]

Rogue also prides itself on its moral authority, claiming that it is part of what it identifies as "The Industrial Revolution 2.0," in which labor and materials are sourced locally, people are paid a fair wage for their labor, and this, in turn, cultivates a thriving local economy and community:

> The Industrial Revolution 2.0 is something we take a tremendous amount of pride in at Rogue. Our mission early on was as much philosophical as it was anything else. Since day one, we have worked to source locally whenever possible. . . . When reading about any product on the Rogue site, we encourage you to look for the "Made in the USA" logo.
>
> We strongly believe that manufacturing creates an ecosystem that is unlike simply a service economy. Workers that earn a fair wage, in turn, have the ability to purchase more goods within that same ecosystem, bringing orders back into factories and sustaining the cycle. When we started Rogue in a garage, we really had no idea just how far we could go. The investment has always been in great people and new equipment.
>
> The Rogue mission really is pretty simple when it comes to principles, but it's also not the "easy" way—otherwise, everyone would be doing it. What good thing ever came easy, though? One step in front of the other, we will take the mountain. See you on the other side.[44]

In a *Men's Health* article titled "The Man of Steel behind CrossFit's Favorite Gym Equipment," Tom Foster enhances our understanding of Rogue and its founder, Bill Henniger:

> Step into your local CrossFit box and chances are you will be lifting Bill Henniger's handiwork. The 44-year-old is the founder, CEO, and sole owner of Rogue Fitness, the Columbus, Ohio, company that makes all the barbells, racks, kettlebells, and other equipment used in most boxes. Henniger was an early CrossFit adopter—he started doing the workouts in 2005 and opened a gym in Columbus in 2007, only to discover that no single company made or sold all the equipment he'd need. An Air Force veteran and General Motors industrial engineer, Henniger fixed that problem by launching Rogue.
>
> He began Rogue as an e-commerce site selling other companies' products and transitioned into making his own.
>
> The company now [2019] employs 600 people in a 600,000-square-foot HQ and buys its steel from American sources. In part, Henniger has set it up that way out of a sense of patriotic duty.[45]

Rogue has a similar origin story to CrossFit: garage-based entrepreneurial endeavors to fill a void in the system, use of the internet and e-commerce, a relationship with the US military, and a strong commitment or patriotism to deeply held values, in this case supporting American families and communities by creating manufacturing jobs and paying a fair/living wage.

According to the *Oxford English Dictionary*, "rogue" is defined as a "dishonest or unprincipled person" or someone "whose behavior one disapproves of but who is nonetheless likable." "Rogue" is also defined as someone who "behaves in an aberrant, faulty, or unpredictable way" or something that is "inferior or defective, deviating from the standard variety." These definitions seem antithetical to the way Rogue, the company, regards itself or is known. Rogue is known for its commitment to community, its honest dealings, and its loyalty to small towns and the United States. It is far from "inferior or defective" with regard to its product and production; it has moved from a garage business to outfitting major sporting and fitness events.

So why name the company "Rogue"? Without knowing the background of the equipment company, a colleague and friend who is familiar with my research on CrossFit asked me, "Every video you post to Instagram has the name 'Rogue' on everything. Is this a nod to 'going rogue'?" To "go rogue" means to "behave erratically or dangerously, especially by disregarding the rules or the usual way of doing something." Although I cannot find any source that confirms that this is the underlying meaning behind the company name, it seems to be a better fit for the ideology of the company, to go against the usual rules of US manufacturing and create an Industrial Revolution 2.0. One article from *Fitt Insider*, a website dedicated to "breaking down the most important developments impacting the business of fitness and wellness," links "rogue" with the company's disregard for the usual rules of fitness and wellness business: "As the antithesis to a Silicon Valley startup or newfangled wellness brand, Rogue is refreshingly old school. Free from buzzwords and world-changing hyperbole, the company's mission and reputation are rooted in values that are noticeably absent from the luxury-inspired, pseudo-scientific trends that dominate the conversation around the $4.2T wellness industry."[46]

Although Rogue might be seen as the antithesis of Silicon Valley, perhaps because, like CrossFit, it was not open to venture capitalism, which would extract rent from affiliate owners to increase shareholder profits, it has roots in Silicon Valley tropes of the garage and identifies itself as masculine resistance to "service industry" (read: occupations largely held by women) exploitation. The "rogue" of Rogue and CrossFit is about the military backdrop of the training methodology and the personal genealogies and preparedness of their founders, one who was raised by a rocket scientist equipping the Department of Defense and the other who is taking the mountain and waiting for us on the other side.

Militarized Fitness

The beloved community of CrossFit is also forged on the violence of the US military and the fears of citizen subjects as they use the training methodology to prepare for life, both on the war front and at home, during the war on terror. This link with the military is not uncommon. Throughout US fitness history, the military has loomed large as a reasons for being fit and in strategies for becoming so. Shelly McKenzie walks us through the various fitness trends and their military ancestors and siblings in her fitness history book. One of the key moments is the end of World War II and the beginning of the Cold War, focusing on future generations of soldiers.[47] President Dwight Eisenhower established a presidential council dedicated to enhancing and testing youth fitness, linking physical fitness with the commander in chief and the US military and bringing physical fitness into the national consciousness through school-led efforts. Over the years, new fitness trends would emerge, often associated with the office of the president or military capabilities. For example, jogging became a national pastime, including the formation of jogging clubs like the one established by President Jimmy Carter, which occurred following the publication of the Air Force Surgeon General's book *Aerobics*.[48] Ronald Reagan was on the cover of *Parade* magazine pumping iron, building visible muscles to match his military might. CrossFit is the legacy of these sorts of fitness genealogies. But unlike jogging or Rambo-type muscles, CrossFit prides itself on preparing for a war that could be enacted anywhere at any time.

The anthropologist Joseph Masco argues that following the dropping of the nuclear bombs in 1945, the United States became a permanently militarized society. This occurred as various US institutions—military, industrial, legislative, academic, economic, and popular culture—worked together to shift the public consciousness and public feeling toward war vigilance and preparedness.[49] Following 9/11, the United States became even more militarized, even as the threat transformed from nuclear weapons to domestic airplanes. The war on terror changed the United States from fears of World War III to left-behind backpacks and shoe bombs.

What Glassman identified as CrossFit's ability to prepare one "for the unknown and unknowable" is akin to Donald Rumsfeld's phrase that epitomized the threats of the war on terror, which are "unknown unknowns."[50] This led to CrossFit being wildly popular among military personnel, including and especially members of the special forces. It has even been identified as a "paramilitary community," as it attracts "military personnel to its method and made gym members into military adjacent people."[51] As I have argued elsewhere, the CrossFit community is built on remembering the war dead, elevating one's workouts by modeling them on those of fallen heroes from the war on terror.[52] CrossFit benefited from a society that was permanently militarized and that increased its militarism post-9/11. It provided a way to calm fears of terror by developing bodies and communities predicated on physical preparedness. CrossFit is a workout regimen in which an Everyman/woman can train like a Navy SEAL, ready to scale walls or deadlift fallen comrades on the war front or at home in Brooklyn.

Conclusion

The CrossFit gym is for people training to be ready for unknown unknowns, the workout regimen cultivating military-ready bodies. It is part of the oracle and garage capitalism of the turn of the twenty-first century, in which men could forge rogue selfhoods made possible by the kind of countercultural attitudes of the restless white men before them. The garage gym found purchase on military outposts and at the edges of cities, the "new frontier" of American capitalism. The frontier is a place of boundary and edge that allowed for domestication as well as rebellion. And it is the frontier to which we turn next.

4

CrossFit and the American Frontier Spirit

I walk into my local CrossFit gym, with its open floor plan in an industrial garage-like space, like the ideal CrossFit gym described in the second volume of the *CrossFit Journal*. On the ground are horse-stall mats, recommended by Greg Glassman as the ideal flooring for a garage gym because they are cheap and can protect equipment being dropped during workouts. Bolted in against the cement walls are gym rigs, or racks that attach to the wall and the ground and enable squatting and pressing at various heights and places to attach pull bars, also adjustable to various heights. These rigs run along the long sides of the gym, a dozen squat and pull-up stations in a row. On the far short side are two whiteboards, one for listing the workout of the day (WOD) and its points of performance and the other for scores from each class. Bumper plates (those designed to be dropped from overhead rather than iron plates such as those in most mainstream gyms) are stacked below the whiteboards. Barbells and clips are stowed in each corner. Along the near short wall sit kettlebells, medicine balls, dumbbells, jump ropes, and resistance bands. Stashed away in corner spaces are a few stationary rowing machines (ergs) and Assaultbikes (a particular brand of stationary bike). The main door to the gym is a gigantic garage door, of a size that would allow a semitruck entry into the cavernous space. Outside these outfitted areas along each wall, the dominant layout of the gym is an open floor plan. Most of the equipment is black or silver, except the resistance bands, which are color-coded. If you walk in after a CrossFit class, you are likely to see pools of sweat and chalk dust on the floor, evidence that a brutal workout took place, maybe one that included thrusters and pull-ups. It might smell a bit musty if the garage door is closed due to the weather. People come here to sweat, and it shows.

The CrossFit garage gym has a spartan feel, a wide-open "What do I do in here?" kind of feel if you are used to mainstream gyms with treadmills, ellipticals, stationary bikes, and various selectorized machines. If you enter during a CrossFit class, you will see several people moving through exercises at breakneck speed, sweating and red-faced, chalking up and lifting heavy and crumbling onto the open floor after they finish, leaving sweat angels on the ground as they do. The open space is filled with people, not machines, during a class. If the garage door is open during the class, a passerby can look in and see the choreographed dance of a CrossFit class during the "MetCon," or metabolic conditioning, portion of the class. It is like group fitness studios in mainstream gyms. However, there are no beautiful wooden floors or mirrors on the walls. Instead, black horse mats, black rigs, and unpainted concrete walls with a garage door to the outside let anyone peer in and witness the spectacle of CrossFit fitness.

CrossFit gyms are built on the garage myth—an open-floor-plan canvas ripe for individual creativity, an undomesticated space filled with masculine bravado, a place for revolution and ingenuity, a temple to the rugged individual who can create or build in such a defiantly barren place. In chapter 3, we considered the role of the garage in American capitalism, especially as it relates to the entrepreneurial spirit. Its position as an undomesticated space near the single-family home also indexes another American myth: the myth of the frontier. Like the garage, the frontier is a place. Like the garage, it is also mythologized and given cultural significance. The frontier serves as "shorthand symbols of patriotism, democracy, rugged individualism, and a host of other virtues," including masculine bravery, vigilante justice, redemptive violence, and an inner moral righteousness based on living in and civilizing the promised land.[1]

CrossFit is in many ways akin to the Wild West or the frontier. Glassman is a "rabid" libertarian, a political position fiercely loyal to frontier ideology: minimal state intervention, an abundance of freedoms, and a sink-or-swim attitude. The affiliate organization of CrossFit is also rather frontier-like; one does not need a lot of capital, just a willing spirit and some moxie. The actual gym space is also akin to the frontier: spartan, minimalist, focusing on "functional" movements and body weight. The ideal body is forged doing pull-ups and squats, not knee extensions on a fancy machine. The ideal community is a bunch of people believing in this ideology. CrossFit is also tightly linked to the US military, which was forged during settler Christian colonialization of the natural environment and Indigenous people. More so, CrossFit is linked to the special forces of the US military, those individuals (almost exclusively men) sent out to get the job done, the tip of the spear with lots of latitude. While no one really talked about the "Wild West" or "the frontier" in the CrossFit gym, it oozes with frontier ideology and a Wild West attitude. It is thus useful to examine the framework of CrossFit as a spartan place for real, "functional," and special forces fitness and the role of the American frontier ethos, spirit, and myth in the production and success of this framework.

The American Frontier

The mythology of the United States hinges on the idea of the frontier and Manifest Destiny, or westward Christian conquest as ordained by God. During the colonial period, much of the westward expansion was curtailed by the British due to fears of costly, violent expansion into Indigenous territory or that claimed by the French.[2] After independence, President Thomas Jefferson doubled the size of the United States with the Louisiana Purchase of 1803. He funded the Lewis and Clark expedition from 1804 to 1807, which resulted in knowledge about the geography and resources of much of the continent.[3] This new knowledge helped facilitate a more popular call to "go West." From 1839 to 1845, the author and editor John O'Sullivan wrote about the United States' divine destiny and coined the phrase "Manifest Destiny." Manifest Destiny was the call to white men to explore, settle, and take the West, to realize the greatness of the US in the name of Christianity:

> The far-reaching, the boundless future will be the era of American greatness. In its magnificent domain of space and time, the nation of many nations is destined to manifest to mankind the excellence of divine principles; to establish on earth the noblest temple ever dedicated to the worship of the Most High—the Sacred and the True. Its floor shall be a hemisphere—its roof the firmament of the star-studded heavens, and its congregation a Union of many Republics, comprising hundreds of happy millions, calling, owning no man master, but governed by God's natural and moral law of equality, the law of brotherhood—of "peace and good will amongst men."[4]

At the same time, Jeffersonian democracy, which required land ownership for voting rights, was giving way to Jacksonian democracy, the suffrage of most white men regardless of land title, forever linking American westward expansion with notions of popular democracy.[5]

As noted by Lewis and Clark, natural resources were abundant in the West, but there were significant impediments to westward expansion despite divine destiny, most notably Indigenous people and lack of infrastructure. Therefore, those who were willing to "go West" required more than divine inspiration; they required bravery, ingenuity, and the will to enact ruthless violence. From 1845 to 1896, the continental United States was forged through settler violence, wars, treaties, and the steady push westward by people seeking a different, better life.

In 1893, Frederick Jackson Turner published a now famous essay, "The Significance of the Frontier in American History," and he would go on to change the way historians, US presidents, and everyday Americans think about the role of the frontier in American life. In that essay, he argues that formally, per official census practices, the frontier is a "line" based on population. On one side of this line are people and civilization, and on the other is wilderness. "America"—its institutions and people—was forged on that line, delicately balanced between civilization and wilderness.

The frontier line was always changing, pushing past the current known white settlement into the wilderness soon to be settled and pushed again. This means the frontier was not just "the Wild West," although that did come to shape the American imaginary and take on significant meaning, but whatever was just west of the current Christian colonial settlement. First, it was New York and the Catskills, Virginia and the Carolinas and the Appalachians. Then it was the Ohio Valley, Tennessee, and the Great Smoky Mountains, then Illinois and Kansas and the Great Plains, and finally past the Great Rocky Mountains and the California and Northwest coast. Thus, the frontier line encapsulated all the United States and created an American spirit of pushing just a bit farther into the unknown, of braving the wilderness.

According to Turner, the pioneers or settlers, those who lived right at the line but on the side of civilization, best represented the American "national character." The pioneers settled at the line, were overtaken by the wilderness, and therefore had to abandon known customs and institutions. Through perseverance and adaptability, the pioneers would overcome and establish themselves, thereby illustrating to others that it was safe and that settler Christian colonial civilization could flourish there. It was through this process that a variety of people from different nations could somehow emerge as "American." It was through the frontier that many ways became one.[6] It is not coincidence that the idea of "whiteness" emerged at this time, in opposition to Indigenous people already inhabiting the area; the shared identity of many European settlers pushing forth became one "American settler."[7] The myth continues in framing these Americans who kept pushing the line west as individually driven; emigration was not government directed. Therefore, those who pushed the line were courageous, individualistic, and prone to egalitarianism, as the frontier required ingenuity, skills, and bravery, not titles or courtesies. The settlers were the embodiment of the American Dream, people investing in their own exceptionalism to push the frontier line ever westward as they settled, planted, and grew their fields, families, and communities.[8] Turner wrote, "to the frontier, the American intellect owes its striking characteristics," including "perennial rebirth," "fluidity of American life," "expansion westward with its new opportunities," "continuous touch with the simplicity of primitive society": "[the frontier] furnish[es] the forces dominating American character."[9] The frontier shaped what it means to be American: rebirth, new opportunities, dedication to freedom and individualism, the valorization of inquisitiveness and bravery.

There have been revisions to Turner's theory over the decades. One of the most prolific historians of the frontier is Ray Billington, who argues that while Turner got a lot wrong, he also got a lot right. Turner was wrong about the processual nature of the frontier turning into civilization: it never worked as seamlessly as he proposed. Fur trappers, speculators, cattlemen, and what Turner and Billington called "Indian fighters" were as present along the frontier line as settlers were. Land was not as cheap or "free" as Turner speculated, so it was not easy for poor city dwellers to head west during economic downturns. Rather, various kinds of people from divergent backgrounds made up the frontier community, often moving west during prosperous times and funded by speculators. Finally, while being ruggedly individualistic, frontier folk had community-oriented views as well. Together, and only together, could they harvest all their crops and build cabins, roads, and schools.[10] These frontier outposts operated as a cooperative of rugged individuals, which facilitated local governance and democratic tendencies.

This is a very idyllic and whitewashed notion of the process of settlement and civilization. The settler life and frontier outposts were also very dangerous and violent. Billington writes that the frontier blends two different images: one pictured it "as a transplanted Eden, overflowing with the bounties of nature and beckoning the dispossessed to a new life of abundance and freedom," while the other painted it "as lawless, brutal, and repelling, molded by a savage environment that reduced the frontiersman to semibarbarism."[11] The settler Christian colonial agenda was met with fierce opposition by Indigenous people throughout the country and particularly around westward expansion. Violence and vigilante justice were also part of the frontier. In fact, for many people, it was as significant as the frontier line.

Violence and Frontier Heroes

Theodore Roosevelt, an avid frontiersman himself, who used his experience in North Dakota to transform himself from a sick boy to a stout man (not unlike Glassman), built on Turner's understanding of the frontier. While not a historian, Roosevelt was a prolific writer at the turn of the twentieth century and focused significantly on the meaning of the frontier as a myth-ideological system to understand the cultural, political, economic, and social systems in the United States. Roosevelt disagreed with Turner on where the frontier began. Whereas Turner thought it was just on this side of the line of civilization, Roosevelt thought it was on the side of the wilderness. Furthermore, in his multivolume treatise, *The Winning of the West*, Roosevelt proposes that American identity and character were indeed forged in the wilderness or the frontier, but they were embodied in the "hunter/fighter," not the settler. The hunter lived well beyond the frontier line rather than settling just before it like the pioneer. This hunter/fighter was the hero winning the West, from animals, Indigenous peoples, and natural wilderness forces. The hunter myth goes as follows: "reared in the forests' haunting silence, these 'primitive-strong' . . . blended the best of primitivism and civilization. Cruel they were, for they must kill the Indians who blocked their countrymen's path westward, but their cruelty was transcended by an inner nobility, a God-given nobility, the gift of intimacy with the Creator through his creations."[12] These mythologized noble hunters were the first heroes in American society who learned the ways of the wilderness (or Indigenous ways of living on and with the land) but also used these violent ways to make way for white, settler Christian colonial expansion.

The cultural historian Richard Slotkin has written three volumes detailing the way the myth of the frontier has shaped American culture and society. All three of them focus on the violence of the frontier. The first examines the Christian myth of regenerative violence as foundational to American life, chronicling American literary culture from 1600 to 1860. The second volume examines the brutality and fatality of the environment during the Industrial Revolution, from 1800 to 1890. Finally, in *Gunfighter Nation*, Slotkin begins with Roosevelt's frontier thesis in the 1880s as the way to "win the West" and concludes with Reagan's presidency in the 1980s and his embodiment—literally—of the cowboy actor coming to power. The myth of the frontier, he argues throughout the three tomes, has transformed throughout US history but has maintained a stronghold on national ideology and narrative about what it means to be American and, more importantly, an American hero, as embodied by the white, Anglo-Saxon, masculine, Protestant hero mobilizing violence to redeem the dream of America. He agreed with Roosevelt, not Turner, in that the "West was won" by hunter-heroes, through violence and the narrative of "redemptive sacrifice."[13]

Despite their differences, Turner, Roosevelt, and Slotkin understood the "frontier" as the most significant force shaping "national character." These ideas—of a frontier, a frontier spirit, the link between the frontier and (white) American identity and national character—were not just the content of historical essays or multivolume treaties. They were the content of the American hero. Long before the comic book superheroes, the men and legends of the Wild West were the American heroes to idolize, including Roosevelt.

Roosevelt played a significant role in frontier mythology. He not only wrote prolifically about his time in North Dakota as a pioneer and cattleman and had his own frontier thesis, which was that violence won the West, but he was also an American frontier hero as the leader of the First

United States Volunteer Cavalry. Roosevelt, an aristocrat, was serving as assistant secretary of the Navy when the United States declared war on the Spanish, today known as the Spanish-American War, after which the US would extend its empire to Puerto Rico, Guam, Hawaii, and the Philippines. Roosevelt resigned from his post as assistant secretary of the Navy and formed a voluntary cavalry from cowboys, Native Americans, small-town sheriffs, and other frontiersmen, as well as city police officers, elite college athletes, and even some men from high society.[14] These men were personally selected by Roosevelt for their adventuring spirit and demonstrable riding and shooting skills. He was named lieutenant colonel of this unit, which became known as "Roosevelt's Rough Riders." Using Roosevelt's influence as assistant secretary of the Navy and as a member of the American aristocracy, the Rough Riders were outfitted with special cowboy-like uniforms and Colt revolvers, the Wild West weapon of choice, and Colt-Browning machine guns.

Roosevelt and the Rough Riders were known for their battle in Cuba against the Spanish army. Seriously outnumbered but rigorously trained and highly resolved, they took, according to legend, San Juan Hill in Santiago de Cuba and planted their cavalry flag. Roosevelt borrowed the term "Rough Riders" from Buffalo Bill Cody's Wild West show, which was popular entertainment at the time. The Rough Riders are one of the most famous examples of US military glory and bravery under fire. They also serve as a precursor of contemporary Navy special forces units, the SEALs, which also embody the tenacious hunter-hero of the American frontier and are connected to CrossFit.[15]

The heroes of the American frontier, much like the myth itself, borrow from legend as well as real life. Roosevelt was a real man who formed a voluntary cavalry. However, the Rough Riders' horses never made it to Cuba, so they fought on foot. And they may not have been the first to take San Juan Hill (some historians believe it was African American Buffalo Soldiers who did).[16] Nonetheless, the legend that they were tenacious fighters who were outnumbered and outgunned lives on.

Another frontier hero is Davy Crockett, a real-life militia colonel who represented Tennessee in the US House of Representatives before dying at the Alamo. He morphed into the legendary "Davy Crockett, King of the Wild Frontier" through his pre-comic-book almanacs in the mid-1800s and Disney portrayals. These men with their legends and their military commands influenced later American military heroes, such as SEAL Team 6.

Superman, Captain America, and other comic book heroes emerged in the late 1930s and '40s, as did the special forces units of the US military, which took shape during World War II. These heroes resemble the frontier heroes; they were marked by rugged individualism, enacting vigilante justice outside of social institutions. They were individuals willing to commit ruthless violence to ensure the safety of humanity or Americans. The American military hero is molded on the hunter-hero as epitomizing the frontier characteristics of American culture. The enemy has changed, but the hunter-hero, with his use of vigilante justice or violence, has remained.

One of the most significant aspects of the frontier thesis is its staying power. Turner's frontier thesis shaped university history departments throughout the country, and Roosevelt (and the traveling entertainment shows of Buffalo Bill Cody) established American heroism and military legends based on this frontier thesis. Slotkin argues that the myth of the frontier has been mobilized by progressives and conservatives, by political managers and movie scriptwriters, by academic historiographers and bureaucratic apologists, and in actual warfare and child's play warfare.[17] The idea of the frontier and its heroes has been ubiquitous to American understandings of itself, its history, and its cultural values. The frontier thesis remains significant, hundreds of years after "the West was won," as a key element of American identity and fantasy. This idea of the frontier, of what the frontier means, remains as an afterlife of what it means to be American. It is an underlying code for understanding how something like CrossFit can become so popular. CrossFit taps into the meanings of the frontier—not because the frontier thesis is correct but because it is the story we tell about ourselves and of our heroes.

A Rabid Libertarian and a Former Navy SEAL: CrossFit's Frontier Spirit

Part real man and part legend, Greg Glassman embodies much of the frontier spirit. In a video by ReasonTV posted in 2013, he claims to be a "rabid libertarian," and he defines this as "not being told what to do." He shares that this libertarian spirit led him to "break free" from the prevailing norms of the mainstream gym's economic and physiologic models and establish a gym and fitness method that could be "raced," where gym members would leave ranked first, second, or eighth after the MetCon. This, he says, "brought a different kind of person around." That kind of person was Greg Amundson, a Santa Cruz deputy sheriff, who says that after one workout with Glassman, "I knew he had the holy grail to fitness, and I never looked back." Another CrossFit coach echoes Glassman and Amundson: "The whole CrossFit political view, it's definitely rogue, it's definitely libertarian. It definitely goes against the norm, against the man, like 'screw the machine,' all that sort of stuff." With this political stance comes a distinct "character" in that "different kind of person," a character who, according to Glassman, is "rough-edged and authentic," "with a mind-set that anything that's worth achieving will come with a substantial sacrifice and commitment with blood, sweat, tears, and other bodily fluids."[18] As mentioned before, a Green Beret told Glassman that the camaraderie of CrossFit was similar to the US Army special forces group forged on agony and laughter.

In the short ReasonTV video, we see the frontier myth, CrossFit edition. A man out west broke free of conventional fitness economic and physiologic institutions and forged his own way. He put up an outpost, and local sheriffs and special forces members, or "a different kind of people," found their way to him. They soon realized that this was the way, and it was predicated on being rough-edged, authentic, and willing to make violent sacrifices to prove their character and win "against the man." While the frontier looks a bit different, the afterlife of the myth remains; the frontier is fitness, and CrossFit, as Rogue claimed in chapter 3 and Roosevelt claimed of the Rough Riders, will take the mountain.

In addition to Greg Glassman, there are other key members of CrossFit HQ who also embody the rogue present-day frontiersman, including and especially Dave Castro. Whereas Glassman walks with a limp due to a childhood bout with polio, is pot-bellied, and is never seen doing a workout himself, Castro is CrossFit's very own Navy SEAL. In a *Men's Health* interview, Castro told the journalist Michael Easter that he started CrossFit as an active-duty Navy SEAL in 2005 and was hooked. The Navy had stationed him in Monterey, California, close enough to drive to Glassman's original CrossFit gym, where he began volunteering.

Within seven months, he was hired on. Today, and for most of his career at CrossFit, he reigns over a hilly sixty-five-acre ranch near Aromas, California, complete with a warehouse filled with squat rigs, barbells, med balls, rowers, and more. The CrossFit Ranch was the site of the first CrossFit Games in 2007. Castro molded the company alongside Glassman, translating Glassman's fitness formula into CrossFit daily workouts (WODs) on the main webpage and public displays in the CrossFit Games. Castro is the director of the Games but is also widely considered the architect of the CrossFit ethos.

This ethos is part libertarian and part hard-core Navy SEAL. It is all white male bravado forged at the California ranch, emblematic of white men with a chip on their shoulders, hellbent on sticking it to the man. These men are modern-day frontiersmen, pushing boundaries of fitness and economic strategy, living lives that are part legend, part real-life hero, and cussing at, spitting on, laughing at, and getting in anyone's face if they disagree. One could not make up caricatures of living hunter-heroes that so match the frontier spirit understood by Roosevelt and Slotkin if one tried. But the frontier is not just forged by hunter-heroes; yes, they are the tip of the spear, but they are not the pioneers or settlers who form the frontier outpost communities. If Glassman and Castro are the hunter-heroes or the tip of the spear, then the CrossFit affiliates, the local gyms, are the settler outposts.

The CrossFit Gym as Frontier

CrossFit gyms are spartan, with horse-stall mats (to be able to drop the barbells), squat racks, and pull-up bars (or simply referred to as "rigs" in CrossFit gyms). They do not have televisions or air-conditioning. As we have seen, they are in garages, and used tires are flipped for exercise. Natalia Petrzela calls the CrossFit gym the "anti-gym" in her book on the history of fitness, because it focuses so much on not being a typical gym with lots of machines, fancy accessories such as saunas, or members who get on cardio machine for hours.[19] There are thousands of CrossFit gyms in the United States and worldwide. As noted earlier, they have often followed the US military to outposts in Baghdad, Qatar, and Afghanistan. But even the local ones, including the ones in New York City, perhaps as far from the frontier as one can imagine, come off as frontier-like. Take one in Brooklyn. According to its website, this is its origin story:

> [We] started in November of 2007 in a small park below a subway line. After three months, we developed a small crew of five to eight people who trained together on the weekends. A fast-approaching winter forced us to find a space we could rent by the hour so we could continue teaching classes and growing the business. We ended up at The Brooklyn Lyceum, an old bathhouse, where we slowly went from two classes per week and about 10 members to classes five days per week and about 50+ consistent members. Many from that crew are still with us. We learned plenty of lessons through a trial-and-error approach as we found our voice as a gym and community. A little over a year later, we moved into our current facility just a few blocks down the street [in an industrial part of Brooklyn]. We [as a community workout] schlepped our equipment over and have been steadily building our program ever since. In 2014, we leased a 1,200 square foot annex space above us for additional offerings and in 2015 we expanded into a second location across the street, which gave us an additional 5,000 square feet [of rolled-up-garage-door industrial space] to accommodate our growing membership and array of class options. Today, we are one of the largest and most well-known CrossFit affiliates worldwide. [The "Our History" section ends with promotional material.] You can see a little slide show of our growth over these past 15+ years on an Instagram highlight set here.[20]

In this commentary, this CrossFit gym reveals its CrossFit and frontier bona fides. It started in a wilderness—outside, in a park, under a subway line—before it had any official space to call home. It then moved to an empty bathhouse/abandoned building, an outpost but at least a settlement. Then, with community cooperation akin to a cabin or school building in the original frontier settlements, the gym moved into an industrial space with a roll-up garage door, tall ceilings for ropes, and an open floor plan. As in the frontier model, more people settled at the initial outpost (former bathhouse), and, after trial and error, it soon found itself "civilizing" into a formal gym space / not an abandoned building. After several years of developing itself, the itch to move, expand, "go west," or colonize more land took over. In classic frontier style, it moved farther into the frontier and settled more industrial space.

However, most CrossFit gyms, even if they do not expand, never quite become "civilized" in the classic gym sense. There will never be mirrors, fancy locker rooms, saunas and steam rooms, televisions for extended time on the cardio machines, air-conditioning, or most of the other accoutrements of mainstream gyms. That is just not who they are. They are the rogue, the outsider, the outpost. They are the open floor plan, the garage, the horse-stall mats, and defiantly barren interiors. In fact, like Brooklyn, the city might grow up or gentrify around the "industrial park" CrossFit gyms, leaving them less on the frontier line and more on Main Street. But the ethos of the frontier remains. They prepare their athletes for the unknown unknowables through functional fitness movements done at high intensity. They demand blood, sweat, and tears from their athletes as much as they provide community and support in the process, building their frontier settlements on the ideals of Green Beret camaraderie, agony, and laughter. One of the most important and "Rough Rider" ways they do this is through Hero WODs—workouts named after US soldiers who did their CrossFit workouts at military outposts in Afghanistan and Iraq and died during their deployments in the war on terror.

American Violence

Slotkin argues in his three-volume history of American culture that the United States has always been a violent nation; as much as it was founded on principles of "religious freedom," such freedom was found behind a weapon, especially the American Colt revolver (created in 1832), which was designed to kill many people at one time. But even before such a weapon was created, conflict and violence were understood as central features of American settler Christian colonialism. The preceding explanation of the frontier thesis includes jobs beyond that of pioneers, including "Indian fighters," which really meant "Indian hunters." To make way for Manifest Destiny, the newly suffraged white men needed to be violent. The historian of the West W. Turrentine Jackson wrote that two elements of the frontier myth dominate: "the equation of masculinity with lawlessness, violence, repulsiveness, and savagery on the one hand, and on the other the myth of the Garden of Eden, the land abundant with resources of nature ripe for exploitation, the gateway to material wealth, political freedom, and upward social mobility."[21] Both parts of the myth require violence, against land, animals, and people. "The history of the United States is a history of violent conquest. Native Americans, Africans, and Mexicans suffered military slaughter, social domination, slavery, and genocide," all at the end of the gun.[22]

Violence was understood as necessary and the purview of the white male to dominate "unoccupied hostile land" and secure his social dominance. The sociologist George Lundskow argues that any threat to white men's social dominance taps into their existential threat of terror, which fuels resentment and rage and thus justifies violence; he calls this the "resentment and terror thesis."[23] This thesis argues that the mere existence of racialized non-Christian Others invokes a terror response in white ethnonationalists but is also a feature of the dominant American white masculinity more broadly. This terror-and-resentment response is historically situated within the frontier mythology and revealed in virtually every mass shooting, as well as the January 6, 2021, storming of the US Capitol. This terror and resentment justifies the use of violence against the Other, using it to "restore" proper social order, "where even the most common man can rise to heroic exaltation with some grit and a gun."[24] This is what Slotkin identifies the US as: the "gunfighter nation."[25]

Historians, anthropologists, and sociologists who study life following the colonial and frontier eras have also found that the United States has always been a violent or at-war nation. And this violence has always been justified by Christian notions of white racial supremacy over Indigenous or non-Christian "heathens." This is true for the settler Christian colonial agenda that ravaged Indigenous people across the continent and allowed for the frontier process to happen. If the "American national character" is predicated on the frontier, then this means that the national character accepts the inherent violence necessary for westward expansion, or the white male Christian imperialism that so defines the United States of America.

American violence has been framed as "defensive." Settlers were defending their communities from the violence of Indigenous people, from the British, from fellow settlers in a lawless land. Violence by the "hunter-hero" made way for the families of settlers to come after them; it protected others. But, as Lundskow illustrates, the fear of others' violence is a projection that Others will be violent, but in reality, it is the settler who was violent. This was articulated well by the anthropologist Joseph Masco, who argues that the US's dropping of the nuclear bombs in 1945 mobilized the US public's affective and imaginative infrastructure toward vigilance and war preparation. In a similar "defensive" strategy, Americans and the US became obsessed and fearful that the bomb, which it had used against Japan twice, would be used against itself. Its own use of violence projected onto the Other evoked paranoia, vigilance, and nationalism.[26]

An afterlife of these historically constituted feelings was their transmutation into terror following the attacks on September 11, 2001. Though I would certainly not argue that the attacks on 9/11 were justified or, in conspiracy theory fashion, the work of the US government, US foreign policy in the centuries and decades preceding the attacks provided context for the events; they were not ahistorical. The United States' violent Christian imperialism throughout North America, Central and South America, the Caribbean, Southeast Asia, the Pacific, and the Middle East reveals the United States' historical practices. The US has not simply been a passive bystander or innocent victim to others' violence but an enactor of violence, often framed as justified, defensive, or holy, since its inception. This is part of our mythology and our reality.

The definition of the nation-state is the authority to take life, to kill. This authority is often enacted by "the law," the justice system, and the military. But the frontier heritage of the United States opened up space for nongovernment officials or everyday white men to "take the law into their own hands" in the form of vigilante justice. The vigilante is predicated on the "hunter-hero." Western lore and legend have been composed mostly of vigilante justice, in which a vigilante saves the community from the corrupt lawmen or Indigenous people. Even modern-day heroes follow the script of the vigilante. The myth of the vigilante is that he is righteous in his violence. The US military is also mythologized as being righteous, despite the reality of what the war machine and warfighter are supposed to do: enact violence. But the military and the vigilante (sometimes within the military) are American heroes, forged through the terror of the frontier and mobilized in the United States' most recent war on terror.

As we have seen, CrossFit has become a popular training method for the US military, local law enforcement and emergency personnel, and even members of the special forces. Part of the popularity of its method with these groups is that it "brings in a different sort of person." The person who is called to CrossFit is one who likes to be ranked, wants to be ranked on achievement rather than on heritage, and finds affinity with the agony and laughter camaraderie of the Green Berets. Those who are called to CrossFit also value its core elements of being constantly varied, high intensity, and functional. Do you want to be able to pull yourself up a rope or over a wall? Do you want to be able to heave heavy things and sling them over your shoulder? Do you want to be able to do such tasks together with others and under the pressure of a clock? Would you not want to use these skills in real life? These aspects of CrossFit have tended to appeal to the military and its personnel.

CrossFit's Militarism and Hero WODs

Military, law enforcement and first responder communities were amongst the earliest proponents of CrossFit. Their intensity matched with the fitness CrossFit provides is a match made in heaven. When a service member dies in the line of duty, a CrossFit hero workout is created in their name. Hero WODs are an opportunity to reflect on the sacrifices of the fallen—to speak their names and honor their memories. These workouts have been a tradition of workout gyms since 2008.
—*CrossFit Journal*

Greg Glassman was invited to give a talk to the United States War College in January 2009. He begins by saying that it is an extraordinary honor to be there and that "there's no audience more important" to him, his program, his staff, and his family. He is even wearing a tie, which, he says, has not happened since 1992.[27] In this speech, he argues that, unlike sport preparation, in which you know the event and the opponent and have maybe even studied video of the opponent, which results in few surprises on game day, the soldier does not get to size up or study their opponent. Some of his first clients were cops and firemen, who were largely confronted with "unknown and unknowable physical challenges" in the line of duty. Therefore, he created CrossFit and the focus of "working on weaknesses" that is inherent to the regimen to help them become better at all kinds of physical challenges, to make the unknowable knowable. Glassman uses examples given to him: the artilleryman needs to be strong to do his job and is thus, presumably, already strong. He needs to work on his weakness, presumably his endurance; the infantryman needs to go long and thus perhaps already excels at endurance. He needs to work on his weakness, presumably his strength and speed. By doing this through the CrossFit model, which is designed for general physical preparedness, they are training for the unknown and knowable.

The US military is full of CrossFitters. Members of the special forces have been known to work at HQ, serving as a bodyguard for Glassman, as the pilot of the company plane, or as the director of training and the CrossFit Games (Castro). The US military uses CrossFit on bases on the home front as well as in outposts and bases across the world. Members of the military do CrossFit, own CrossFit gyms, and even use CrossFit to help them reenter society following deployments. In a 2023 article in *Reserves + National Guard*, two reservists are highlighted. First is New Jersey National Guard Captain Ellia Miller, who once hated exercise but, after finding CrossFit, was hooked. She says, "With CrossFit, you're training your body to do anything you might need to do within a combat role or whatever else you need to do in the military."[28] Miller has competed in the military division of CrossFit's annual Occupational Games, earning the title of "Fittest Military Service Member" twice. Navy Reserve Petty Officer First Class Alexander Spears did not play sports as a child and never considered himself an athlete. Then he found CrossFit during a deployment to Afghanistan when the base gym hosted classes. He, too, became devoted.[29]

While I have not been in all US CrossFit gyms, it would not be a stretch to say that every one flies an American flag or hangs one on the wall. Next time you enter any gym outside of CrossFit, see if they have as American flag hanging. Some CrossFit gyms, especially those that are veteran owned, hang flags representing the various branches of the armed services. Much like Roosevelt and his Rough Riders planting the cavalry flag on San Juan Hill, CrossFit plants the American flag in each gym to represent the claim that the US armed forces, service members, and the nation-state have on that land.

One of the most notable elements of CrossFit is its Hero WODs. "Since 2005, CrossFit has posted workouts meant to honor the memories of CrossFit service members who made the ultimate sacrifice and exemplary members of the CrossFit community who are no longer with us."[30] Hero WODs are officially named CrossFit workouts begun in 2005 and established as "tradition" by 2008. They are almost always named after a white male US soldier (occasionally after a firefighter or CIA agents, like "The Seven") who has died during the war on terror. To create a Hero WOD, one emails CrossFit with the specifics of a workout and the information about the soldier who died—his rank, where and how he died, and who survives him. There are almost two hundred Hero WODs. On the CrossFit Hero WOD website, each workout is accompanied by a photo, most depicting the person in military gear, field camouflage, or dress uniform. Murph is one of these Hero WODs and arguably the most "famous" one.

The Murph Hero WOD was created in 2005 following the death of Navy SEAL Lieutenant Michael P. Murphy of Long Island. He lost his life during a SEAL mission to capture a Taliban leader in Afghanistan. He and the team had been trapped in a firefight behind enemy lines, needing to call Bagram Air Base for backup. Murphy abandoned cover to make the call and was shot. Murphy was awarded the Congressional Medal of Honor in 2007 for his bravery and sacrifice. A Hollywood movie was made about the lone survivor of the mission. According to the CrossFit website, "This workout was one of Mike's favorites and he named it 'Body Armor.' From here on it will be referred to as 'Murph' in honor of the focused warrior and great American who wanted nothing more in life than to serve this great country and the beautiful people who make it what it is."[31] The favorite "Body Armor" workout—one-mile run, one hundred pull-ups, two hundred push-ups, three hundred squats, one-mile run, with a weighted vest—is now "Murph." All hero WODs are like this, named after the fallen soldier and based on a favorite workout of theirs.

One of my first weekends conducting research on CrossFit happened to be Memorial Day, the "unofficial" beginning of summer in the US, as the holiday falls in late May. A common way to celebrate this holiday honoring fallen US soldiers is to have picnics, cookouts, maybe a parade, or perhaps a local 5k run. This is a typical way to recognize those soldiers who have paid the ultimate sacrifice for their country and for "American freedoms." These traditional activities are the official stories (NNP) of Memorial Day, and most Americans can tell you them if you ask.

"Murph" is done in most CrossFit gyms in the United States on Memorial Day. At the CrossFit gym I observed, Murph's information, where he was from, his rank, and how he died, was shared by the CrossFit coach before each group fitness class began the Memorial Day workout: Lieutenant Michael Murphy was killed on June 28, 2005, during Operation Enduring Freedom in Afghanistan. He was twenty-nine. He was a lieutenant in the SEALs. During his life, he called this workout "Body Armor."[32] He performed this workout in Afghanistan, in one of the military-CrossFit-gym outposts. I have watched hundreds of people do some sort of variant of Murph: those in weighted vests, those who scaled the volume of the workout, those new to CrossFit, and those who had done it almost a dozen times.

Josh Appel, the leader of the Air Force pararescue team that rescued the survivor and recovered those who died, reflected about doing Murph on Memorial Day, "It's not just about Michael Murphy. It's an opportunity to memorialize everybody that's paid the ultimate sacrifice. Instead of going out and having a barbecue, go out and suffer a little bit and think about sacrifices people have made.... You put out a little pain, a little blood, a little sweat, some tears, for them."[33] Everyone I have observed do Murph was dripping sweat, breathing hard, and red-faced. They sprawl out on the concrete outside the gym's rolled-up garage door after they finish the final mile. Everyone was sore in the days after. If you are not, you did not quite do it right. And most CrossFitters do it right. That is part of the ethos. There are standards, and one of them is to go hard and push yourself past your limits, like Michael Murphy.

I have written about my own experience doing Murph as I tried to make sense of the ritual of doing workouts named for dead soldiers as a way of honoring them and building community.[34] Ultimately, CrossFit gyms organize an event that honors US soldiers, sharing the holiday with family and friends over food and drink. Yet there is something meaningful in that the event is not a nonspecific "5k" but rather "Murph," the name of a specific Navy SEAL, and the event is his favorite workout.

What does it mean to do a workout named after someone who is dead? What does it mean that it is called a "hero" workout? How is this different from a 5k? Is it important that the "body armor" did not save his life? The meaning that inheres in CrossFitters performing Hero WODs is that they are not just a Memorial Day 5k. Doing Murph is an American-made, frontier-forged, military-tested, and "Built Ford Tough" fitness endeavor. CrossFit and Hero WODs are the embodiment of America at its finest, fittest, and toughest, even though it is dead war fighters/warriors who provide the branding.[35]

But CrossFit is not just about honoring war dead; it is about preparing the living for battle. Major Lisa Jaster was the third woman to become an Army Ranger, graduating from Army Ranger School in 2015, the first year women were allowed to enroll. She credits CrossFit for her success. CrossFit prepared her not only physically for the grueling fitness tests but also for the mental ones, including being away from her children, including a three-year-old, for six months. Despite her earning her "Ranger tab," she could not apply for the Seventy-Fifth Ranger Regiment, like the male graduates, because the regiment, along with many other special forces, was closed to women then.[36] This changed in 2017, when the Seventy-Fifth Ranger Regiment made history as the first special forces unit to allow entry to women.[37]

CrossFit also created CrossFit Defense, a special training course that combines constantly varied functional movements performed at high intensity with a "lightning-fast, genetically ingrained method of self-protection."[38] CrossFit Defense prepares the CrossFitter physically and mentally for being ambushed by unleashing what Tony Blauer, the creator of CrossFit Defense, calls everyone's "completely natural, subconscious, lightning-fast, tactical human weapon system."[39] Humans, according to this view, are naturally weapons systems, and CrossFit Defense helps unleash that power; it is especially useful for police tactical units, special forces personnel, or elementary school teachers who want to survive a school shooting.[40]

The "American-made" heroes of the WODs and the use of CrossFit to prepare for special forces entry (especially for women) or to prepare for ambush violence are linchpins in the success of the CrossFit fitness regimen and brand. They tap into the frontier or wilderness, which demands that one develop capacities that are not required for civilized life but that are necessary in a violent world. They are about "functional fitness" and "intensity." In the context of the rugged individualism of the United States, CrossFit and Hero WODs call to everyday Americans to build their own capacities as weapons systems to become "harder to kill."[41]

Conclusion

CrossFit's link to the frontier is obvious in the gyms, the Hero WODs, and the relationship with the military. CrossFit's ideology and culture valorize violence, battle, the US military, the special forces, law enforcement, and anyone who wants to survive gun violence. To emphasize this point, on July 13, 2016, Dave Castro, the Navy SEAL and CrossFit Games director, announced that the winners of each division (male, female, team) would be awarded a Glock pistol for being crowned the "Fittest on Earth." While many CrossFitters petitioned not to have a handgun as an award for the Games winners, Castro held fast.[42] And all of the winners were white. The very same day as Castro's announcement, LeBron James, Carmelo Anthony, Chris Paul, and Dwayne Wade—four Black National Basketball Association (NBA) superstars—took to the stage at the ESPY Awards, an annual award ceremony for ESPN, and pleaded for professional athletes to do something to end gun violence.[43] As the religious studies scholar Rachel Wagner writes, "Guns are made for ending things. . . . The gun is a sacramental object which binds the gun holder to an imagined, imminent future in which violence is the means to a good life. Guns become a ritualized way of asserting dominance, and a means of imagining oneself tasked with saving the world."[44] The scholar and activist Roxanne Dunbar-Ortiz says that although "nearly anything, including human hands, may be used to kill, only the gun is created for the specific purpose of killing a living creature."[45] The awarding of the gun to white winners of the CrossFit Games stands in stark contrast to the Black NBA players calling for the end to gun violence. CrossFit embraces the mythology of the gun, its specific purpose for killing a living creature, and the need to survive gun violence rather than strive to end it because its training method and brand are linked to frontier values, "defensive" white violence against others, and gun glory.

Everyday CrossFit is linked to the frontier myth. Gyms are often established in industrial areas of town, away from Main Street or the commercial area. In its defiantly barren, wide-open space, real exercise can happen; people can lift heavy and burpee fast, together in a competitive spirit. I imagine if Frederick Turner were still alive, he would think the CrossFit gym was the pioneer of the fitness world, staking claims on health and community on just this side of civilization. Roosevelt might identify the role of the Navy SEALs and the Hero workouts as evidence that CrossFitters are the current embodiment of the hunter-hero, not the pioneer. Either way, the CrossFit gym as a settler gym or the CrossFitter as hunter-hero training like a Navy SEAL or the third female Army Ranger taps into frameworks of the frontier and thus provides a way for everyday (mostly white) Americans to live out an American hero journey or lifestyle.

5

Heroes and Sheroes

[What is CrossFit?] It's a community of dedicated fitness practitioners. I don't know that I have a better answer. . . . The impact that the affiliates have on their clients in the gyms is exactly who we are. I cannot believe how many 21, 22, and 23-year-old kids come up to me and get it all. They get the opportunity for them as young affiliates. They get the uniqueness of the physiological adaptation. They get the uniqueness of the business model. They get the no rent extraction commitment on our parts. . . . They're fans of everything we do, and they're just *quiet heroes* in their own little community.
—Greg Glassman, *CrossFit Journal* (emphasis added)

Last summer the finals of the CrossFit Games were broadcast on ESPN. Forty-five thousand people showed up to watch the contestants who look like *superheroes* heave, jump, and lift until a champion was crowned.
—Sharyn Alfonsi, in the *60 Minutes* segment "King of CrossFit" (emphasis added)

The five of us, all white women in our early to late thirties, are headed to a local powerlifting competition on the other side of Brooklyn. They let me tag along. I had only been observing at the CrossFit gym for a few weeks, but the powerlifting coaches, who coached both CrossFit and specialty powerlifting classes, had made a point to include me in their activities. One named me "the Margaret Mead of the Meatheads." They extended an invitation to all training sessions and competitions, such as the one we are driving to today. The five of us are all wearing our gym's T-shirt, a version of the sports jersey or a Christian pilgrimage badge one can buy at each affiliate to index fandom, to go cheer on another friend who is competing.

"So how is the transition?" Monica, the driver, asks Talia, who is sitting in front.

"Well, I couldn't be happier." She turns around to look at me, as I am the only one who does not know: "I recently gave up my law practice to become a CrossFit coach and to do the nutrition courses to become a nutrition coach. I am getting divorced because my lawyer husband doesn't understand why I would do such a thing. But I'm dating another coach who does."

I am a bit shocked at such a major life overhaul, but I manage a nod and a "How did that happen?"

"I just couldn't manage both—taking care of myself and being a junior lawyer. I don't want to spend my life in an office, sitting at a desk. So yeah, changing jobs and getting divorced!"

"I've noticed your traps [trapezius, neck muscles]! You are doing something right!" Heather comments from the back seat. "You can always tell a woman who does CrossFit by her traps."

Talia laughs. "Thank you. There is also that. I stopped fitting into any of my work clothes." Her newly built muscles have made her lawyer attire, suits, and nonelastic fabric too tight around the back and shoulders. I could not help but think of She-Hulk, her muscles busting out of her lawyer clothes. "I'm a bit nervous about it all. But I also haven't felt this good in years, so there's that. Speaking of, how's the new nutrition stuff going, Mon?"

Monica is trying to get pregnant, and one of the recommendations is for her to cut down on sugar, including alcoholic beverages. "I am drinking those waters that are sweet like crazy," she laughs. "It's been tough. I'm just more tired and cranky. But the end goal is worth it. [My coach] has changed some of my programming too, to accommodate the reduction in carbs. I mean, I feel better and know it is better for my health, but sometimes I just want that donut!"

"I hate cuts!" Heather chimes in again. She has competed in powerlifting more than anyone else and has "cut weight" to be able to compete in her preferred weight class.

"I haven't done one yet, but [Coach] thinks maybe for State's. The lower [weight] class is way less competitive," Danielle, the woman to my right, adds. She has qualified for the New York State Championships in powerlifting and has a better chance of medaling (being top three) if she cuts to a lower weight class.

"Are you already counting your macros? Make sure you get one to one and a half grams of protein per pound of body weight. If you need any help, I'm happy to do your nutrition coaching for free while I train in the new program," Talia offers Danielle.

"I'd love that. I need all the help I can get."

"We should also ask [Coach] to organize another clothing swap. I have a lot of stuff that could use a good home. I will be wearing Lulu for the foreseeable future! Fingers crossed [new boyfriend] can help me become an ambassador for them, like he is," Talia laughs. I think of Superman exchanging his office attire for his blue spandex and red cape. Talia is not going back to pinstripes; she is sticking with the athleisure tights and hoping to be sponsored by the local Lululemon store. This sponsorship would include a giant mural of Talia and her muscles on the wall of the store, as if to say it is the clothes that made this superwoman's body.

* * *

This was the first time in my research that I had heard someone mention career and marriage changes due to CrossFit. I had read about them—the lore is like Talia's experience. People find CrossFit, and it changes their life, so much that their previous major life decisions do not "fit" anymore, like clothes purchased before their bodies had muscles. Instead, they find new meaning and life partners at the CrossFit gym. Talia was the first person I knew in real life who had made such dramatic life changes. She would not be the last. The clothing swap was real as well, indexing a metaphorical meaning: everyone would bring in the clothes that no longer fit, and everyone would look through everyone else's closet to find something new. People swapped out new clothes and new lives at the CrossFit gym. Talia swapped out a career in law for a career in fitness and nutrition; she swapped out her sedentary lawyer husband for a fit coaching boyfriend. She was moving out of her old home and into her new boyfriend's digs the following weekend. Swapping one for the other, hoping she did not hurt too many feelings (her parents', her ex's, those of the other women at her gym whom her new boyfriend had dated) along the way.

This was also one of the first conversations I could follow about nutrition. The language around food was much different in the CrossFit gym compared to mainstream fitness venues I had been in. People did not talk about "diets" or "calorie counting" as much as they talked about "cuts" (or "bulks") or "macro counting." Macronutrients (fats, carbohydrates, and protein) and their relative distribution in one's diet was how people learned to think about food, rather than calories. Macro distribution shaped getting bigger or smaller and was about building muscle rather than only weight-on-the-scale changes. This way of talking about food and nutrition was about preparing the body to do heroic things, such as lift as much weight as one possibly could one time, do challenging CrossFit workouts for time, or build a fertilized egg into a human being.

During this short car-ride conversation, it was obvious how normal conversations about major life changes were for these four women. Bodily changes, which included increased muscle mass or biochemical conditions for pregnancy, were everyday conversations. Life transformations were commonplace thanks to new practices and relationships found at the CrossFit gym. Swapping clothes or men, careers or donuts, powerlifting medals or body weight was part of the new bodies and lifestyles that these women were forging at the box. CrossFitters, both men and women, were using an exercise practice and the community of others to forge new bodies and lives. To use Glassman's words in the first epigraph to this chapter, they were quietly becoming the heroes in their own lives and communities, busting out of old clothes and lives to reshape who they are and with whom they built a life. They were on their way, if they worked hard enough, to looking like superheroes like the CrossFit Games athletes.

As we have seen, Hero WODs bear strong links to the frontier thesis that established important American cultural values and ideology and the brand of the American-made hero: the wake of the hunter-hero and vigilante has since informed other forms of hero iconography, including the Navy SEAL but also comic book heroes. Yet the American idea of heroism extends beyond the frontier legend, into the mythology of the hero and his journey. This idea also links back to the CrossFit heroes—the superstars and the everyday CrossFitters, including the women who do CrossFit. Building on the example of Army Ranger Lisa Jaster, we can see how women who do CrossFit at various levels feel "empowered" in their lives through the training methods to become a particular masculine version of a female-hero (shero).

The American Hero's Journey: The American Monomyth

In the psychologist Carl Jung's quest to find the "collective unconscious of humanity," he examined myths, symbols, and stories from peoples around the world to see how they overlapped and what, if anything, might be universal.[1] He argued that there are twelve "archetypes" that are manifested in "all cultures." These include the Mother, Shadow, Wise Man, and Hero. The Hero overcomes obstacles and achieves certain goals that require courage and perseverance. The psychologist Joseph Campbell took up the mantle of the universal unconscious and argued that there is one (mono) universal story that each human culture uses, while modifying it to create its own unique variation. He called this "the monomyth" and posited that it undergirds every cultural mythology. He sought to prove this theory in his book *The Hero with a Thousand Faces*, with an examination of various myths of "the Hero," arguing that they all were fundamentally the same. He compared "the hero" in Christianity, Greek mythology, Egyptian theology, African Yoruba religion, European folk tradition, Native American spirituality, Islam, and many others. On the basis of this cross-cultural analysis, he argued that there is a universal "hero's journey." In this "hero monomyth," the hero is called to adventure, faces and overcomes obstacles, comes to understand something important, atones and transforms from these experiences, and returns home to share his new and hard-won self with his people.[2] The narrative structure of these myths is one of separation, rite of initiation, and reintegration as a new, better man. Campbell argues that this myth and its narrative structure are universal.

Much like the example of the "redemptive self" discussed earlier, some scholars argue that there is an American cultural story of the hero that differs from the universal one. John Shelton Lawrence and Robert Jewett are two of the most prolific scholars on the American hero who argue that there is an "American monomyth" that diverges from Campbell's universal model. The American monomyth goes something like this: "A community in a harmonious paradise is threatened by evil; normal institutions fail to contend with this threat; a selfless superhero emerges to renounce temptations and carry out the redemptive task; aided by fate, his decisive victory restores the community to its paradisiacal conditions; the superhero then recedes into obscurity."[3] In contrast to the "classical monomyth," which, they argue, reflects rites of initiation, the American monomyth derives from tales of redemption. "It secularizes the Judaeo-Christian dramas of community redemption that have arisen on American soil, combining elements of the selfless servant who impassively gives his life for others and the zealous crusader who destroys evil."[4] This American hero monomyth has "historical, philosophical, and theological origins in a variety of factors surrounding the founding and development of the United States, especially puritanism, liberal Protestantism, frontier expansion, Western literature, national independence from England, and cultural separation from Europe in general."[5]

Lawrence and Jewett trace this American superhero monomyth throughout American popular culture from its birth in the colonial era (harmonious paradise of early Christian America) to Buffalo Bill Cody (frontiersman) to superheroic/lawbreaking vigilante presidents (George Washington and Abraham Lincoln) to Disney characters to *Star Wars* and *Star Trek* heroes to *The Matrix* (Neo) to military heroes (Rambo) and Captain America and his "crusade against evil" in the post-9/11 United States. They argue that these heroes and their tall tales continuously remind Americans what it means to be an American hero, replete with underlying codes of violent redemption grounded in white masculine Christian ideals.[6] In another book on superhero comics and theology, the scholar of theology and culture Anthony Mills argues that American Christian theologians and comic books, especially the Marvel ones by Stan Lee, were "saying things about what it means to be human in late-modern American culture, . . . and they were largely saying the *same* things."[7] The cultural historian Sean Guynes and the religious studies scholar Martin Lund argue in their book on whiteness and American superhero comics that comic books and the transmedial adaptations of their stories have "transformed the white male body, and the boundaries of morality and justice that it polices and upholds, into a widely circulated visual lexicon of white (male) superiority."[8] The American hero is a white selfless (Christian) crusader whose (frontier-forged) vigilante actions are acceptable to save the paradise that is America from villains (people of color, women, nonheterosexual people, differently abled people, immigrants, poor people, and so on) wishing to destroy it. This story of white male American righteous vigilante heroism is the ubiquitous stuff of popular culture and real-life heroes.

It is no coincidence that the rise of the current deluge of superhero movies emerged in post-9/11 America. Ten superhero movies came out in 2019, the most in a single year. But nine were released in 2008, 2016, and 2017, eight in 2018 and 2021, six in 2005, 2011, and 2014, and five in 2004.[9] That is seventy-six superhero movies since 2004. Ronald Reagan once stated that his viewing of Hollywood films probably shaped his military policy; perhaps he is not the only one.[10] These films and their narratives permeate popular culture, shaping ideas of what it means to be American and a superhero: a white man with extraordinary physical and mental abilities.[11]

CrossFit emerged in the post-9/11 world, becoming popular through training newly enlisted soldiers, members of the special forces, returning veterans, and nonsoldiers who wanted to train like a Navy SEAL to embody the American hero. CrossFit tapped into the new post-9/11 world of anxiety and fear of real-life villains, and it mobilized a deeply entrenched hero story in its boxes, workouts, and ideology. Superheroism in CrossFit is not left to the storybooks or the cinema screen. Superheroism is embodied by those who perform the workouts. It is the rigorous enactment of a superhero lifestyle; it is daily gym training for unknown unknowns (or, if you do it right, unknown knowables). It is the building of one's internal "engine" to perform feats of strength, endurance, power, agility, and balance. It is the building of muscular bodies through exercise and nutrition to look like those of the cinematic or CrossFit Games superheroes. CrossFit encourages everyday people to train like Navy SEALs, like CrossFit Games athletes, to build their bodies so that their muscles bust out of their law-office clothing and to forge a community of like-minded others who want to do the same. It wants people to become the "quiet heroes" in their own communities. It is the forging of communities of quiet, heavily muscled or "jacked" heroes who train and build every day just in case "shit hits the fan" like it did on 9/11 or other dire events, and they can save the day.

CrossFit Heroism

Three forms of heroism are enacted in CrossFit. The first is the most iconic or ideal: the CrossFit Games athletes who are crowned the fittest people on Earth. These individuals look like they are carved from marble, the living, breathing heroes from the movies. The second is the CrossFit gym that swoops in to save the day when members need support. And the third is the everyday CrossFitter—here we will focus on women—who forge empowered senses of self through their training. However, this new, empowered sense of self is built on "masculine" attributes including strength, muscles, entitlement, and rugged individualism.

CrossFit Games Bodies as On-Brand Hero

Unlike for viewers of the superhero movies or costumed fans at Comic-Con, the American hero moves from the screen or costume to the body for CrossFitters through CrossFit's rigorous training. While all commercial fitness sells a "better you," CrossFit pushes the "onus of the brand onto the body itself," requiring "a deeper commitment to the routine, including dietary changes, clothing or gear that in some way manages discomfort, and advice sought from teachers or coaches instead of medical professionals."[12] The body forged through CrossFit is visibly muscular and is also capable of heroic acts, those necessary for military deployment, hand-to-hand combat, or winning the CrossFit Games. CrossFit bodies are billboards for a particular heroic lifestyle forged in the CrossFit gym.

Every year, usually in February, Dave Castro directs the CrossFit Open, which leads to the CrossFit Games. The Open ranges from five (in 2017) to three (in 2024) weeks of workouts, each week's workout revealed on a Thursday night as a livestream event of elite CrossFitters are pitted against each other to show how it is done. Every CrossFitter can sign up to participate in the Open, with affiliates encouraging everyone to join. Participation for the Open peaked in 2018, when 415,000 people participated worldwide. The Open is an online qualifier to the next stages (Regionals or Regional Qualifiers), with each stage whittling the field until eighty meet up to compete for the title of "Fittest on Earth" at the CrossFit Games. If one is not a member of a box, one can still participate by posting one's workout videos and times online. While the Open is more participatory and anyone can "play," as the numbers are whittled down to forty men and forty women, the cream of the CrossFit crop rises, and similar-looking athletes find themselves qualifying for the Games: very muscular white men and women. According to Sharyn Alfonsi on *60 Minutes*, they look like superheroes.

A quick Google search for "Superman" produces images of Christopher Reeve (1970s) and Henry Cavill (2010s), both visibly muscled white men, with dark hair, piercing eyes, and a strong jaw. But one quickly notices how much more muscularly defined Cavill's Superman is than Reeve's. Cavill's Superman is jacked, his deltoids and pectoral muscles more pronounced. Cavill's Superman looks more like a CrossFitter than Reeve's; this is due to CrossFit-style training. Cavill used the same fitness trainer, Mark Twight at Gym Jones in Utah, who trained Gerard Butler and the rest of the Spartans in the movie *300*.[13] (Gym Jones was originally a CrossFit affiliate, and many of the workouts Twight uses are CrossFit style; but there was a falling out with CrossFit.) Video of Cavill training for his Superman role has him in a garage gym deadlifting, Olympic lifting, and using gymnastics rings and other equipment made popular by CrossFit and Rogue.[14] Functional fitness methods helped Cavill bulk up for his über-muscular and defined version of Superman.[15]

CrossFit women have also been perceived as superhero-like. It is common knowledge in CrossFit gyms that many of the women in Wonder Woman's Amazonian army in the 2017 Warner Bros. film were CrossFitters, already-muscled women plucked from the CrossFit Games roster to play superheroes on the big screen.[16] Wonder Woman did not have the muscular build of a CrossFit Games athlete, but the all-woman tribe of superwomen did. Twenty-first-century Superman and the Amazonians of Wonder Woman look a lot like an elite CrossFit Games athlete.

Real-life elite CrossFit Games athletes include Tia-Clair Toomey, Annie Thorisdóttir, Sara Sigmundsdóttir, Katrin Davidsdóttir, Rich Froning, and Matt Fraser. A Google search will reveal the "look" of these individuals: white, on the shorter side for athletes (five foot four to five foot nine), jacked, and relatively naked. "The -dottirs" (as Annie, Sara, and Katrin are colloquially called) are all from Iceland, white, blond, five foot seven, and visibly muscled. Rich and Matt are blue-blooded

Americans, former college baseball players a bit too small for Division I sports or the big leagues. Tia is a white Australian who represented her home country at the 2000 Sydney Olympics in weightlifting. Except for gymnasts and figure skaters, short stature can be an impediment to professional sports. Even the average height of the Navy SEALs, still an all-male unit, is five foot eleven, well above the elite male CrossFit Games participants.[17] In the sport of fitness, height privilege, which is the improved status afforded to those who are taller, is inversed.[18] Average American height (five foot nine for men, five foot four for women) is considered acceptable, if not preferable, for those competing to be "Fittest on Earth"—the Everyman or Clark Kent who, with a change of clothes, can become a superhero or Superman.[19]

What these elite CrossFit athletes lack in height, they make up for in their muscular physique. Compared to most other sports—basketball, soccer, baseball, even American football—CrossFit Games athletes are more muscularly developed, akin to elite sprinters and gymnasts. During CrossFit—at the Games or even during workouts at the affiliates—muscles are on display. CrossFit is known for its "barely there" uniforms: men without shirts and women in short, tight luon shorts and sports bras, which reveal rippled abs on both men and women. Superhero physiques, like Cavill's in Superman or Gerard's in *300*, were developed by a commitment to CrossFit. These are the bodies of elite CrossFitters: white, short, attractive, jacked, and somewhat unclothed. Both the sport and the business/brand of CrossFit and of the American superhero traffic "almost exclusively in heteronormative Whiteness."[20]

The American comic book superheroes, and their cinematic versions, are fundamentally figures of whiteness, predicated on their (white) power and supremacy.[21] Although this may seem self-evident given the prevalence of superhero narratives that center on the protagonists' superior white bodies, Guynes and Lund note that the relationship between whiteness and the American superhero is painfully unexplored.[22] In the two giant tomes by Lawrence and Jewett, they chronicle the Christian roots of the American hero myths in (almost painful) detail. Their texts are a tour de force on the subject of heroism, arguing for the American hero to have its own monomyth. But not once do they examine the hero's skin color or the privileges, powers, and legacies attached to whiteness. There is no mention of whiteness or white supremacy; nothing "white" appears in these books' indexes. Perhaps "Christian" is code for white, or as Toni Morrison is often quoted as saying, "In this country American means white. Everybody else has to hyphenate"—the whiteness of the American hero and superhero is blatantly obvious to anyone.[23] Willie James Jennings writes in his book on Christianity and the origins of race that whiteness is never a surprise but the result of structural thought.[24] "White," "American," and "Christian" are interchangeable terms to mean a particular kind of structural thought. While not all American superheroes are white, the vast majority of those who get to be heroic look a particular kind of way: white and male/masculine, with a moral compass that points to Christianity saving humankind from the terrors of non-white-male Others.

Cody Musselman writes in her work on CrossFit and religion, "The CrossFit brand isn't coincidentally a product consumed largely by white people; it's a product designed *by* and *for* white people."[25] In fact, she writes, a latent social Darwinism simmers barely beneath the surface of the atmosphere, as individuals utter slogans ("Stronger. Faster. Harder to Kill.") and fight for titles ("Fittest Athletes," "Fittest Fans," "Fittest Man," "Fittest Woman") that suggest that a stronger body can be molded through the right disciplined practices, especially if one is white. It was the eugenics movement, which embraced a racist ideology that white people were genetically superior to other "races," that held "Fitter Family Contests" at local and state fairs in the 1920s to illustrate the "superior results" of proper (white, heteronormative, Christian) breeding techniques that would begin the "fight" for "fittest."[26] The body on top of the CrossFit podium is almost always white. Scanning the roster of top competitors and podium finishers, one observes an overwhelmingly white majority. This racial preponderance differs from other sports that include more people of color or where the top finishers are Black. CrossFit superheroes, much like the majority of American (Christian) superheroes, are white.

CrossFit Gyms: Saving the Day

The second hero is the CrossFit gym, often coming to the rescue of its members. In one of my local gyms, a member was diagnosed with cancer, and a GoFundMe was set up by the gym in her name. Within a day, she had exceeded her goal of $30,000, reaching about $200,000 for her medical care and income while she underwent chemotherapy and radiation. Other CrossFit gyms have similar stories. In August 2023, a tropical storm hit California, causing a CrossFit couple's outdoor wedding venue to cancel their event. Their local gym, CrossFit 1886, saved the day by allowing the couple to use the gym. After the 10 a.m. CrossFit class, volunteers from the gym transformed the gym into a perfect wedding space; "the entire community came together to make sure the Evans' wedding was a success."[27] It is common to hear stories about how CrossFit gyms mobilize the venues and members to help out their fellow CrossFitters. Not only do they provide space and a logic for exercise and health, but they also use their membership to help others, from assisting people to move to babysitting services to cancer and wedding support.

One particularly complex story of the mobilization of a CrossFit gym community is that of Atom Ziniewicz, told in the *CrossFit Journal*.[28] Ziniewicz was a veteran Green Beret, a CrossFit athlete, and a CrossFit affiliate owner in Virginia who suffered from posttraumatic stress disorder (PTSD) and bipolar disorder; both diagnoses followed his deployment to Afghanistan and Iraq. During his most intense suffering, his CrossFit gym rallied around him: he found shelter at a coach's house following his marital separation, members were understanding when he failed to show up to coach classes, and after his death, they dedicated an annual regional competition hosted at the gym, called the Cold War, to his memory and raised money for Invisible Wounds, a nonprofit that helps veterans with PTSD, and the National Alliance on Mental Illness. The gym even keeps Ziniewicz's biography on its website in his memory. Ziniewicz suffered immensely after his return to everyday life, and the tone of the story in the *Journal* and of the local affiliate's homage is one of honor and respect.

Ziniewicz's story is more complicated, however. During an intense manic episode, he left Virginia for Alaska, stopped taking his medication, and purchased $400 worth of alcohol from a local liquor store. A man and a woman visited him in his cabin, and though it is unclear what exactly happened, Ziniewicz ended up shooting the man twice before both visitors fled, reported the incident, and sought medical treatment for the gunshot wounds. Alaska State Troopers, Alaska Wildlife Troops, a K-9 unit, and an Emergency Reaction Team arrived at the cabin to find Ziniewicz emerging from the nearby woods. Everyone drew their weapons, and Ziniewicz was fatally shot. The last paragraph of the article in the *Journal* states, "Nobody knows what Ziniewicz was looking for in Alaska, or what he was thinking when he faced down the state troopers. What is clear is that despite the efforts of his friends, his family, and his community, Ziniewicz did not get the help he needed, and he chose the only option he thought remained."[29]

One of the comments posted to the online version of the article reads, "I find it odd glorifying a man who shot another man."[30] In the article, there is a vague reference to the man who was shot being associated with drugs and an indication that no cash was found at the scene, as a way to suggest that the man somehow was deserving of the gunshot wounds; one of the commentors to the article defended Ziniewicz by remarking that the man, who had been jailed for drug offenses earlier in the year, "only suffered superficial flesh wounds."[31]

We see here the unfolding of the American hero monomyth. Recall that this monomyth goes something like this: a community in a harmonious paradise is threatened by evil; normal institutions fail to contend with this threat; a selfless superhero emerges to renounce temptations and carry out the redemptive task; aided by fate, his decisive victory restores the community to its paradisiacal conditions; the superhero then recedes into obscurity. The United States suffered an attack on 9/11 because the "powers that be" ignored dire warnings. Ziniewicz, a brave, selfless man, enlists and sacrifices his youth by going to war. He becomes a Green Beret and serves his country; he returns home to establish a local CrossFit gym beloved by its members. Paradise is restored. But unable to reintegrate into normal social life, Ziniewicz recedes into obscurity. Perhaps this is why he goes to Alaska, the present-day American frontier. He also enacts vigilante justice, like a frontier man, like the original American heroes, and the Every(white)man with a "little grit and gun," against a man who might have stolen from him.[32] Suffering from the terror that justifies frontier violence and vigilante justice, Ziniewicz shoots the man and then pulls his gun on "the Law" and is killed by it. Nonetheless, his CrossFit community continues to uphold him as a hero, exactly as complicated as the American monomyth describes. The idea of forging heroes in the CrossFit gym empowers many to be the hero in their own stories.

Embodying CrossFit: Sheroic Selves in Stronger Bodies

I can lift heavy things. My roommates ask me to do the grunt work around the house. People, men usually, are always impressed when I throw the cafeteria tables around at school, etc. I am fit. I look fit. I work hard to be fit. I can't even be self-deprecating or modest about the subject. There is no question that I am stronger and "more fit" than the average Joe *and* Jill.
—Sophia, a thirty-year-old white K–12 teacher

During my research in the summer of 2017, the CrossFit Games was shown on a large screen at the CrossFit gym during our daily workouts. The women on the screen were referred to as "Greek goddesses" or as "#bodygoals" by my fellow Brooklyn CrossFitters. None of us looked like that; but they were the ideal, and their bodies provided inspiration for what we could do and look like if we dedicated enough to what Coach called "sweat equity" (hard work in the gym) and "dietary considerations." We needed to show up and push ourselves in the gym, go heavier in the strength portion, or go faster in the MetCon portion of the workouts. We needed to properly fuel for the workout and the recovery. We needed to drink enough water, get enough sleep, and quit alcohol—all of us: men, women, and children (recall Marcia and her entry into CrossFit at age nine).

In the quotation that begins this section, Sophia exemplifies the payoff if one follows inspiration with "sweat equity"; she can lift heavy things, the telltale sign of the CrossFitter. Talia, whom we met earlier, has changed her body, especially through the building of trapezius muscles, another sign of a CrossFitter. She has also transformed other embodied experiences, including her intimate life and her professional life, to better adhere to CrossFit. She has changed jobs (from lawyer to CrossFit and nutrition coach), has changed lovers (from lawyer to CrossFit coach), and is dedicating her life to CrossFit through her embodied choices of diet, career, and family. Sophia, Monica, Heather, and Danielle have all mobilized CrossFit-led diet, exercise, and coaching to change their lives in very intimate ways. They do not just wear the gym's T-shirt; they literally use CrossFit to transform their bodies, as revealed through muscle gain, fat loss, or pregnancy. They have all committed to CrossFit's promise of a "better self," revealed through the transformation of the body, and even to transformations of personal, intimate, and family lives. In this process, they come to feel empowered, the hero in their own stories.

Despite our discussion of superheroes, people in CrossFit do not go around talking about the frontier, superheroes, or being a hero, at least not in any explicit way. They talk around it. They reference pushing their limits and getting better. They discuss hitting goals, getting stronger, and gaining visible muscle. Related ideas come across when they talk about WODs and having survived them, especially when "getting through" them is more challenging than they initially thought. Sometimes the daily workout requires a deep commitment and/or a heroic belief in one's abilities.

Take, for example, Sophia. Sophia told me about what CrossFit means to her and how her life has changed since starting it. She does not mention being a hero, but reading her words, one gets the sense that she is proud of "what she is capable of" thanks to CrossFit and her new, powerful embodied self forged in the CrossFit gym:

> I've seen the most dramatic transformation since the start of the year.... I've always eaten healthily, but dialing in my nutrition and being more precise about what I'm eating and how much has really made a difference. Now I can *see* all those muscles I've been building.... I can definitely see muscle development in places like my shoulders and back. At first, it was a little alarming, but I think that's because women are so conditioned to think that skinny/small [equals] beautiful. The truth is, I've never had that body, and CrossFit has helped me accept how I'm built and actually really optimize it. I can honestly say today that I'm proud of this body and actually love a lot of things about it, which is a pretty big deal for me.
>
> I'm incredibly inspired by the amazing, beautiful, *strong* women at this gym and in this space in general. I read something recently on the blog about how women's bodies are typically judged based on what they look like rather than what they are capable of and that this totally sells us short and holds us back. CrossFit helps you build a body with purpose and function, and I think that's incredibly empowering—for everyone but women especially! I love how CrossFit really flies in the face of a lot of the common tropes/trends/myths about women and fitness.

What's so great about CrossFit is you're constantly getting to experience that high of hitting a goal. Heavy lifting and Olympic lifting in general, pull-ups, toes-to-bar, and kipping pull-ups are all highlights of the last year. But what's so fun is there's always something new to accomplish! I also feel like simply committing to a super-disciplined workout routine that I stick to religiously is a milestone.

I truly believe the confidence I've gained in the gym has made me better at work. . . . I'm more inclined to speak up, lead, and take on challenges. And in general, my workout routine helps me manage my stress and mood swings better. I just love being pushed and challenged.

I believe 100 [percent] that CrossFit has changed my life. It's affected how I view myself and what I'm capable of, which has reverberated in my career and beyond. It's renewed my sense of discipline. And it's given me a new passion in life!

Sophia's story is emblematic of those of other women I interviewed at the gym. She does not call herself a hero, but she talks about cultivating a way of life and a self that she is proud of, finds ways to push through really challenging workouts, which prepares her for life's craziness and stress, and builds an optimized body and mind through nutrition, training, and rejecting limiting fitness tropes. CrossFit provides a sense of empowerment—to lift heavy, to practice hard things, to set and achieve new goals, to be a person one is proud of.

Sophia's story is reminiscent of Talia's talk about busting out of her lawyer clothing while I imagine She-Hulk as she says it. The muscles these women are building and seeing are the embodiment of their heroism. They represent the other heroic elements that CrossFit has forged in them: speaking up at work, taking on challenges, changing careers or divorcing one's husband, throwing around cafeteria tables, and appreciating a more robust, muscled body as beautiful in a world that asks women to be smaller, to be paid less, to make sensible choices, to take up less space. The bodies these women are forging are reflections of the heroic selves they are cultivating. CrossFit muscles come with confidence. CrossFit stamina comes with moxie.

In addition to Hero WODs that allow everyday CrossFitters to perform their favorite workouts named after real-life military heroes, Cross-Fitters embody these heroic values—stepping out of their comfort zone, facing body pain and tears, pulling themselves together, and never quitting. In addition to the fitness tests or the community-building events based on Hero WODs, everyday workouts allow CrossFitters to forge a heroic self in the daily routine of the gym. Showing up and getting through the daily grind of CrossFit encourages people to be proud of the person they have become.

A fair amount of academic literature on CrossFit focuses on the female bodies of CrossFitters. Many of these studies investigate whether the muscles on these female CrossFitters challenge normative, mainstream, or hegemonic femininity or masculinity in the United States. Many of them focus on the "icons" of CrossFit or the elite Games athletes. The scholars of communications Myra Washington and Megan Economides conclude, based on their analysis of CrossFit media, that "CrossFit expanded possibilities for the female body while continuing to mirror a hegemonic archetype of attractive and heteronormative femininity." They write that elite CrossFit women have the "markers of femininity" in their donning of tight clothing, makeup, and perfectly styled hair. They also have "traditional markers of masculinity such as well-defined muscles, weightlifting accoutrements, and strength."[33] The professor of English Leslie Heywood, one of the most prolific scholars of CrossFit, examined a CrossFit documentary, *Every Second Counts*, that "was instrumental in describing and instituting CrossFit as a sport, and helped to disseminate its central, often contradictory, premises." In this documentary, at the second-ever CrossFit Games in 2008, Glassman told the winner, Jason Khalipa, that he was not "only world champion [but had] a demonstrable, evidenced-based contention for world's fittest human being": "Wear that well—you're the product of [CrossFit]."[34] Khalipa was the fittest human being; women were an afterthought, seen in the documentary as wives or girlfriends in supporting roles, rather than as the Games athletes they were. The scholar of health and sport studies Bobbi Knapp examined CrossFit imagery in the *CrossFit Journal* and interviewed female CrossFitters at a local box, concluding that while the CrossFit images of women ultimately undergird, they also subtly challenge, heteronormative femininity.[35]

CrossFit's popular slogans, such as "strong is the new skinny/sexy/beautiful," "both challenge traditional gender norms and reinforce hegemonic conventions, as they place a demand on the female body to be strong while remaining traditionally appealing."[36] The culture and media studies scholars Riikka Turtiainen and Usva Friman analyzed images and media presentations from the 2019 CrossFit Games, concluding that there is an ambivalence to women's strength and dominance in performance even at the Games level. For example, during the broadcast of the Games, whenever a woman's strength was discussed by the commentators, the camera would cut to images of her distinctly cultivated heteronormative femininity, including long hair, pearl earrings, mini shorts, and sports bra.[37] In addition, women's dominance over men resulted in male athletes being shamed for losing to a woman rather than praising the woman's win. For example, there were two events that demanded an equal workload for men and women (not often the case due to various CrossFit standards), and women outperformed the male athletes. Turtiainen and Friman conclude, "Instead of celebrating the female athletes' strength, the attention and shame are directed at the male athletes beaten by the women. After all, even though the female athletes (and everyday CrossFitters) are encouraged to compete at the men's level, women are never supposed to actually win."[38]

Women are not supposed to win because CrossFit traffics in hegemonic masculinity. Hegemonic masculinity's features include power defined by physical attributes like a strong, tough, capable body. That powerful body dominates men, women, and children while also being heterosexual in its desires. Hegemonic masculinity also means high achievement in work, sports, or other avenues and being a daring or rugged individual; it is a romanticized version of the frontiersman.[39] In the linguistics scholar Victoria Kerry's autoethnographic and semiotic analysis of a CrossFit gym in New Zealand, she examines the myriad ways hegemonic masculinity took hold of her gym and herself. She examines the name of the gym, The Cave, which "is distinctly masculine, despite women having lived in caves as much as men did. [The name] evokes ideas such as 'man caves'—male spaces which women are banned from so that men can get on with their own activities—or 'cavemen,' who dragged women back to their caves against their wills." She observes how the whiteboard is a hierarchy of male achievements, and the Cave Rules of the gym demanded masculine toughness. The gym imagery, such as the Hulk and the gym's logo of a red skull with dripping blood signifying pain, also reinforce masculine ideals, as does gym merchandise emblazoned with pain-glorifying messages such as the women's T-shirt "Harden up, Princess." Kerry even examines her own internalizing of such hegemonic masculine messaging in her commitment to CrossFit and The Cave.[40]

But CrossFit is known for its encouragement of female strength and the embodiment of the brand in muscles or calluses formed in both men and women, and women embody masculine-stereotyped imagery—ripped and enlarged abdominal muscles, enlarged muscles in the neck (Monica and her "traps"), and phenomenal strength in the Olympic lifts—as much as the men do. In fact, without the sports bras, tight mini shorts, pearl earrings, and long-styled hair to indicate one's femininity, elite CrossFit Games athletes' bodies, male and female, would look very much the same. This is the brand hero of CrossFit—advertised in ideal form in the fittest humans (men and women) on Earth and in the bodies of everyday CrossFitters who strive to look like their gods and goddesses.

Contradictions

On a popular competitive fitness magazine website, Dusan Balaban writes,

> Why are some CrossFit workouts named after girls? According to CrossFit Founder, Greg Glassman, he named the benchmark workouts after girls in similar way that storms are named after girls by the National Weather Service. He felt that, because these workouts are so physically demanding, they leave you feeling as if a storm had just hit you.
>
> [Dusan quotes Glassman's well-known explanation:] "I think anything that leaves you laying on your back, gasping for air, wondering what just happened to you should be named after a girl."
> —Greg Glassman.
>
> The "Girls" refer to a collection of workouts named after women trailblazing in CrossFit. The original CrossFit Girls, introduced in September 2003, were Angie, Barbara, Chelsea, Diane, Elizabeth, and Fran. Helen and Grace were introduced a few months later.
>
> Girl CrossFit benchmark workouts are important training milestones within the CrossFit training methodology. They act as a great way to test

your fitness against your previous self and see how you have improved and developed.[41]

On the one hand, "The Girls" are the first "named" benchmark workouts; benchmark workouts are those done to test one's fitness against others and against a previous self. This use of female names for these challenging workouts appears to be a nod to the equal appreciation that CrossFit is said to have for women's physiques and work capacities. In the United States, mainstream gyms are known for their gendered spaces: women in the cardio or studio spaces and men in the weight areas.[42] Women repeatedly tell personal trainers, "I don't want to get bulky," which means "too muscle-y."[43] Rather, they want to get "lean" or "toned." Women are also told not to lift too heavy, or else their feminine features might "shrink."[44] But CrossFit women—like Sophia earlier—are proud of their muscles and their fitness compared to other men and women, even as they understand this as in contrast to mainstream beauty standards. Their bodies are idolized by other CrossFit women as powerful (and sexy). On the other hand, the diminutive use of "girl" and the lore of the naming—something that has you lying on your back gasping for air must be named after a woman—reveals a sexist element to the naming strategy; a Reddit posts suggests a rephrasing as "Heroines."[45]

But the heroism of women and deep misogyny are not mutually exclusive in the patriarchal United States. This is the law of the frontier, where female pioneers were just as "capable" against the wilderness as their male counterparts were. Think sharp-shooting Annie Oakley. It is how Wyoming became the "Equality State," allowing women suffrage before any other, as they were already leading homesteads, facing a wilderness, and "winning." Similarly, CrossFit heroism can include Hero WODs and The Girls, women with bulging muscles throwing equipment around in their day jobs, Greek goddesses on the competition platform, and women who are fitter than most "Joes *and* Jills." They are building themselves to be American heroes, "Ford tough." And they are developing their genetic potential in ugly, barren gyms where the barbell becomes a friend, squats reveal character, paleo/caveman diets allow for extended training, and forged muscles reveal that if they lived a million years ago—definitely the wilderness—they would not be eaten. But they also should be pretty, with their hair and makeup done, in tight-fitted clothing, and wearing some pearl earrings.

In all this hero talk and body talk, one figure is glaringly absent in the videos of workouts, or on the podium of the Games, with his shirt off revealing his eight-pack. Many wonder what happened to Greg Glassman, the founder of this embodied regime, because he does not ever do the workouts and he does not have a "CrossFit body." In fact, he walks with a limp due to childhood polio and has a potbelly under his CrossFit T-shirt. He does not have visible muscles; it does not look like he even works out, let alone is committed to his hero-building fitness regimen. In the comment section of a *CrossFit Journal* article from January 2010 titled "You Are CrossFit," someone writes, "How come Coach doesn't do the WOD at these events? Is there a reason for that? Are there any videos on this site [CrossFit.com] of Coach doing a WOD, it would be cool to see the founder of CrossFit doing a workout. I've searched and haven't found any."[46]

The very next comment reads, "Hahah [name of author of the above comment]! Careful..." A handful of other CrossFitters reply, some sticking up for Glassman and saying he would do the WODs if he wanted to, others chiming in that it would be cool to see Glassman do his own regimen, especially when CrossFit claims to be accessible to all because of each workout's scalability. Still others told this commentor not to "ruffle any feathers." But this commentor writes that he is genuinely interested in why "there is no evidence of Mr. Glassman showing us how to do a WOD" and that if folks think he is "ruffling feathers than [sic] you need to ask yourself why the Emperor has no clothes."[47] The comment section devolves from people discussing why they, the everyday CrossFitters, "are CrossFit" (the original journal article theme) to why Glassman should or should not do his own workout regimen. One comment seems to sum up most of the others with the following: "There are very few people that I regard as highly as Greg Glassman. I consider him to be a great American, the archetype of a hardworking, self-reliant, rugged individualistic patriot."[48]

There does not need to be evidence of Glassman doing a WOD or of his muscled body. Even without muscles or other proof of fitness, Glassman embodies the ideals and values of CrossFit by making the regimen itself, gifting the training method to the masses, and leading a revolution from his oracle perch in his garage. He is the archetype of the white, masculine American hero, rogue and ready for a fight.

Conclusion

It is the elite CrossFitters on the podium who inspire dedication to the regimen as heroes full of muscle and strength. But it is in the local gyms where heroism is exemplified. Owners and members are the "quiet heroes," as Glassman calls them in the epigraph to this chapter, who financially support friends with cancer or prepare the barren garage space to host a wedding. They are the Sophias and the Talias who transform their lives with their commitment to CrossFit. They find meaning in the regimen and community and find confidence and muscles through their dedication. In many cases, these elite and local CrossFitters reflect the American superhero monomyth: white, masculine, courageous, and yet a bit unable to satisfy stereotypes of proper man- or womanhood. Therefore, they forge ahead as a "new super breed," created by Glassman: part Rocky Balboa in *Rocky IV*, created in a spartan garage/barn by tapping into a primordial human past, and part Ivan Drago in *Rocky IV*, built using cutting-edge scientific claims. We turn to the scientific claims that build the superhero-CrossFit body next.

6

Science, CrossFit Style

After the brutal workout, I just wanted to sit down for a little bit. Catch my breath. Let my face lose its tomato coloring. My current gym had a sitting area in the front, with two couches, a coffee table, and a book stand. You could take a book, just bring it back. You could sit on the couch; you just had to fight the gym dogs for a spot. No one seemed to care that the dogs occupied the couches because the people who sat on them were just as stinky, especially post-WOD. Beyond the little living room area, on the back side of the second couch, was a matted floor space. The entire gym was outfitted in the rubber mats one finds at most CrossFit gyms, the kind Glassman says you can get at your local horse feed and tack stores.[1] But this area, between the couches and the actual workout space, is where we warmed up and cooled down, where we foam rolled, used lacrosse balls, and stretched, and where most folks wrote in their journals. The wall behind the warm-up/cool-down area was where the Leaderboard listed all the best times in the gym, the top three men and top three women for The Girls and many of the Hero WODs. It also included the heaviest clean and jerk, snatch, squat, deadlift, and strict press and the fastest one-mile. As we warmed up, we did so under the names of the gym's best.

As I found my way to the cool-down area, I watched as most folks took out a little notebook and wrote down their numbers from the day as they recovered. It was a Monday, which, during this eight-week cycle of programming, meant deadlifts and bent-over-rows. A cycle is meant to increase strength in one area and help measure progress.

During the workout, those of us in the class were summoned to the whiteboard, where the first CrossFit coach gave a minilecture on the "points of performance" of the deadlift: "Barbell over the laces of the shoe, slight bend to the knee, hands outside the knees, brace, and stand it up. Be sure to focus on the hinging of the hips not the bending of the knees." The second CrossFit coach would demonstrate the movement as the first one spoke. The second coach then gave the points of performance for the bent-over-rows. We were to use dumbbells to focus on single-arm strength, stabilizing ourselves with a box or bench. Technique was important, as more weight, fitness experts and coaches argue, can be lifted with proper technique. We were to "superset" these movements: deadlift and then row, for five sets of five each. This should take us fifteen to twenty minutes. All of this is standard knowledge for kinesiologists or exercise scientists.

Because my gym had many members, sometimes our classes had thirty or more participants; we were usually paired up. One of us deadlifted while the other rowed. We were paired up by the coach, who would do so based on our deadlift strength.

"Who is at 315?" the first coach asked. Two of the strongest men raised their hands. They were going to deadlift "three wheels" for five sets of five, an impressive feat of strength.

"275? 225?" and so on down the list. I raised my hand at 185 and was paired up with Ben. We all steadily went back and forth from barbell to dumbbell, working on our strength. After we finished our five sets, we put our equipment away and circled up at the whiteboard one more time for insights into the MetCon.

The MetCon was a 21-15-9 toes-to-bar (T2B) and thruster 95/65 couplet. This means we had to do twenty-one T2B, a skill in which one holds onto and hangs from a pull-up bar and brings one's toes to the bar and then back down—often they are done with a swinging or kipping motion—then twenty-one thrusters, a barbell skill in which the barbell is caught in a deep squat and then it is thrust overhead, then fifteen each, and finally nine each. If one were to do it as "prescribed" or "Rx'ed," then men were to use ninety-five pounds on the barbell, including the weight of the barbell ("men's" bars are forty-five pounds), and women were to do sixty-five (with a women's thirty-five-pound barbell). Of course, one could "scale" the workout. On the gym's webpage under "Workout of the Day," the guidance was, "Scale the Toes-to-Bars to Hanging Leg or Knee Raises as needed to get through the reps in 1–3 sets. The Thruster weight should be on the light-medium side for you and unbroken on the fast end. Post times and Rx to comments." It was being done "for time," or as fast as possible. We were to go as fast as we could; it was a race to finish first.[2]

We all loaded up our barbells, positioned ourselves under a pull-up bar on one of the gym's racks, and waited for the beeping of the countdown clock: "3 . . . 2 . . . 1 . . . Beep!" We all jumped up and did what we could for the twenty-one T2B, followed by thrusters and then back to the pull-up bar for more T2B, and so on. One of the coaches turned up the music before both coaches moved around the gym to watch for standards: Did our toes touch the bar? They had to or they did not "count" if one was Rx-ing the workout. Did our hips go below our knees in the thruster, and did our elbows lock out at the top of the thrust? These are the "standards" of a thruster. We all know these rules. When finished, we collapsed on the ground, and the coach turned down the music.

"Well done, everyone! Be sure to write down your weights and times for today on the board." A queue formed near another whiteboard where everyone who has done the WOD writes down their deadlift weight, then their time, and if they Rx'ed the workout. It looks something like this on the whiteboard: "Katie, 185#, 4:39 Rx." At the end of each day, the gym takes a photo of the whiteboard of scores for posterity.

Some people wrote their information on the blog, as instructed by the webpage. Some blog postings might include more information to be clear and to help those who might do the workout later in the day: "Abby, WOD in 6:29 Rx. (8-7-6/12-9, 3-2-3-2-3-2/8-7, 3-2-1-1-1-1/9)" or "Francis, WOD in 9:13 Rx. First round felt really slow and bad. Took me a minute to get my t2b rhythm right. Tried to hold myself to my rep scheme (7-7-7, 5-5-5, 3-3-3) for the most part, which helped me mentally. And got a great cue from [coach] to hold onto the bar for the last set of thrusters. . . . Powering through those 9 unbroken was the right move!" In Abby's description, we learn how she "breaks up" the repetitions. Instead of doing twenty-one all at one time, she does eight and then seven and then six of T2B and then does the same with the round of twenty-one for thrusters: she does twelve and then nine at a time. During the final set of nine, she is so tired that she ends up doing singles of T2B. We can read into Abby's workout enumeration how hard that workout was for her at the end: she was barely able to do one at a time. Francis writes out how he feels "really slow and bad." He had gone into the workout with a "strategy" of doing three sets of equal repetitions. That "helped mentally" with the difficulty of the workout. However, he was "pushed" a little bit by the coach not to do sets of three but to power through. This choice was "the right move" and undoubtedly helped him finish with a faster time.

After writing on the whiteboard the CliffsNotes version of the times and weights, many folks cooled down while writing in their notebooks.

Ryan, who was sitting next to me, rolling out his lower back, told me, "I am on my fifth notebook."

"Wow! Are you getting any better?" I asked. I thought of one of CrossFit's handful of definitions of fitness: "increased work capacity across broad time and modal domains." Was Ryan's work capacity getting better across broad time and modal domains? Was he stronger and faster at everything?

"Definitely from the first year! It's crazy to look back and remember what it was like to be weak and not know how to do anything. Then it becomes, 'Am I fitter?' Sometimes the answer is no, so you got to up your game." He did not necessarily use a CrossFit definition, but he did use the number of logbooks to gauge his fitness.

One CrossFit gym in Massachusetts provides a common breakdown of why logging workouts is so important in CrossFit:

> Why should you record your score? If you're a member of [CrossFit gym] you're competing. That doesn't mean you're trying to out-run, out-squat, or out-fitness your buddy next to you (although for some it does—and that's okay). It means you're making yourself a little bit uncomfortable, pushing yourself a little more than you'd like, pursuing a little bit of that "better" you've come to expect from the effort you're putting into the workout. In other words, *you're competing against your yesterday self.*
>
> *Recording our scores on the whiteboard creates a sense of community*, a weekly diary of folks who've thrown down and suffered those brutal WODs either next to you, before you, or after you. It can also give you a little bit of motivation.
>
> Recording our scores on the website creates a digital journal that you get to revisit each time we do that workout again. *While CrossFit thrives on variety, we also like to measure our progress.* Writing your workout score on the website helps us measure our progress: Are we getting fitter? Did we move faster? Did we lift heavier? Did we feel better?
>
> To help get you on your "recording" way, we've broken down the recipe to a successful website post. Go ahead, give it a try!

Your Score: Write down your score, your weights, your rep scheme, your modifications. Anything you would need to know to recreate the workout as you performed it. This "should" be a fairly objective exercise.

How did you feel: Record how you felt during this workout. Were you just not feeling it? Were you pregnant? Just add a little color (not excuses) so that you have some context the next time we perform the WOD.

Your strategy: How did you attack the workout? Did you break up the sets in any given way? Where did you rest? What would you do differently next time? This isn't just to "game" the WOD, it's to motivate yourself to work just a little bit harder and more effectively next time.[3]

Even if one does not do local CrossFit competitions or have their sights set on bigger CrossFit glory (such as the Games), the logic of CrossFit is that you are always competing with yourself and sometimes with your "gym nemesis," as one CrossFitter called the guy he "competed" against (had similar numbers to) most regularly. Logging scores on the whiteboard "creates a sense of community," as you know who suffered with, before, or after you in the workout. It also helps the gym owner and/or coaches know if the programming is working. Does Francis power through the thrusters during the last round? Does Abby do more T2B unbroken? Are you fitter than your "yesterday self"? Ryan had five notebooks of his "yesterday selves" in the form of workout times and strength numbers with which to gauge his progress.

A company called Beyond the Whiteboard, or BTWB, was established to fill a need in CrossFit. It is an app that provides a convenient place for gyms and individuals to log their scores and keep track of their training. It connects CrossFitters to others "beyond" their own gym's whiteboard. BTWB allows a CrossFitter to see what their time in a named workout is compared to "hundreds of thousands" of users worldwide.[4] BTWB, like dropping into a CrossFit gym during one's local or transnational travels, allows for CrossFitters to see how they measure up against people doing the same workouts anywhere in the world. As with other CrossFit-inspired companies, it began in 2007 with a couple of friends tinkering around trying to make logging workouts more seamless and individual work more meaningful and to build on their passion for CrossFit to extend the community beyond the local whiteboards. Hundreds of thousands of CrossFitters around the world, like Abby, Francis, and Ryan, log their workouts. Is that not what data is? Is that not what scientists do? Fill notebooks with numbers and data?

One of the more surreal moments in my early CrossFit days was when gym bros, men dedicated to working out and knowing trendy fitness information, began lecturing me on the evolutionary basis and scientific authority of their paleo diet and of CrossFit's functional fitness. "Paleo" they claimed, echoing lectures they had heard from CrossFit authorities, was how humans were meant to eat. Functional fitness—squatting and deadlifting—were how humans were meant to move. Recall Glassman's claim to "deliver" to us our genetic potential, what we would look like "a million years ago." As I am a member of the field dedicated to understanding current humans and human evolution through contemporary primate behavior and the fossil record, it took effort not to provide an Introduction to Anthropology lecture on the inaccuracies of these beliefs. I wanted to remind people that modern humans were not around a million years ago and are built to walk long distances, slowly. I wanted to give examples of the variety of human diets throughout history and geography, evincing that there is not one diet that reveals humanity's genetic potential. But my lecturing would not matter because CrossFit's use of "science" is not simply about the empirical method but about the use of numbers to give an aura of scientific legitimacy and claim authority through expertise.

In examining the logics of science that CrossFit mobilizes to make its claim that it is a superior fitness regimen to others, we can focus on the recording of workout times as a method of audit culture. We can also examine the use of the "paleo diet" and "functional fitness" exercises as a means to scientize the training method. We consider Glassman's weaponization of science, his use of "science guys," and his "math" mind to take on the fitness establishment for their lack of scientific rigor or compromised funding sources. Glassman does this in vigilante-superhero fashion as he and his Army Ranger bodyguard engage in "Battles" for the scientific soul of the fitness industry.

CrossFit Numbers: Science or Audit?

For a nonscientist, filling up notebooks with numerical observations might feel like science. In fact, it was science for much of the past two thousand years, a practice attributed to Aristotle (~300 BCE). The Aristotelian model is predicated on making observations, seeing patterns in these observations, and using these data and logic to propose a theory of what is happening. Much of the approach taken in this book relies on this method, which is termed "inductive" inquiry or research. This method is sharply contrasted with the modern scientific method, which is hypothesis and experiment driven: observe something, wonder about it, formulate a research question and a testable hypothesis, perform an experiment and collect data, analyze the data, make and report conclusions, and then do it again. This is termed "deductive" research, inquiry, or logic: it is focused on testing something (a dependent variable) by keeping everything else the same (independent variables). Deductive work was developed to replace inductive reasoning or logic; it is attributed to Francis Bacon (~1620). Bacon's work was focused on refuting the Aristotelian *philosophy* of natural science with *methodology*.

The difference between these two methods is what differentiates the "social" sciences from the "natural" sciences, the "soft" from the "hard" sciences, and sociology from chemistry. The disciplines of psychology, anthropology, and physics include researchers using each method, with the laboratory factions generally considered more "scientific," while the others are "theoretical." In addition to the differences in these methods of inquiry, there are differences in the social value attached to each. Considerable value is placed on "hard" science as the authority of real knowledge, reducible to natural "law" rather than the product of human observation. Hard science is considered above reproach or incorruptible, simply reflecting nature (Baconian method) rather than relying on human observation and thus individual variation or human error (Aristotelian method).

There has been a turn in American society toward quantification or the enumeration of daily life. This is the transformation of a "daily walk" into "ten thousand steps" or the swapping of "a good night's sleep" with "a sleep score." With this enumeration or quantification comes the aura of science and math. The anthropologist Sally Engle Merry, who examines the enumeration of society, argues that numbers *seem* to be simple descriptors of phenomena, existing outside of bias or theory because they *must be* "subject to the invariable rules of mathematics."[5] There is an assumption that numbers and mathematics are objective. But Merry argues that numbers carry with them assumptions about what *should* be counted (e.g., steps, not the number of trees seen on the walk) and then postulations that such things make up ordered knowledge. This ordered knowledge becomes "calculative rationalities" that are grounded in financial accounting practices. In other words, this is not science; this is accounting.

This counting is what Michael Power has called an "audit system" and is modeled after financial audits and performance measurement systems, which are systems with a knowledge base and a method of scoring or grading.[6] Audit systems have their roots in the enumeration of cadets' activities at West Point Military Academy in 1817. Cadets' lives and the tasks they were supposed to perform were scored, and those with the highest scores were placed in premier positions. This kind of scoring of tasks in the hope of improved performance was refined by Frederick Taylor in his 1913 book *The Principles of Scientific Management*, in which he analyzed workflows to improve labor productivity. Enumeration was not about science; it was about making a more efficient workforce by using principles of accounting. Henry Ford was doing similar things, and his mass-production principles paralleled Taylor's "scientific management." A focus on work and production using accounting principles created task-driven, fiercely competitive environments where the system was gamed for an advantage, including achieving output targets over quality control.[7]

Power wrote two books about auditing: *The Audit Explosion* (1994) and *The Audit Society: Rituals of Verification* (1999). Both examine the proliferation of auditing and audit systems throughout society—in the military, hospitals, education, the nonprofit sector, sports, and so on— to *prove* something through enumeration, including quality, efficiency, or effectiveness. This approach is a distortion of both the Baconian and Aristotelian scientific methods: it involves enumerating desired observations to make them seem more "natural" and to elicit preferred behaviors. It is the widespread proliferation of these calculative rationalities of modern financial accounting and their effects on individuals and organizations that the anthropologists Cris Shore and Susan Wright call "audit culture."[8] The anthropologist Marilyn Strathern also examines auditing, audit systems, and culture. She writes that audit is not focused just on what *is* happening but on what *ought* to happen; it is about en-

hancement or providing a moral code to the measuring at hand. "Audit occupies the modest position of enabler—assisting persons and institutions to compete better" as if in a marketplace.[9] Audit culture was thriving right as CrossFit was coming onto the scene.

Glassman used audit culture to help him define fitness and score workout performance. One of the most important origin stories of CrossFit purports that Glassman was the first to define fitness. As the story goes, in 2002, Glassman read an *Outside* magazine article that identified a triathlete as the fittest man on Earth. Glassman agreed on some grounds: sure, the triathlete was probably a good swimmer, runner, and cyclist. But he disagreed on others: Could he produce power? Was he strong? Was he flexible? Glassman wondered what definition of fitness *Outside* magazine was using if it was going to measure fitness or make such proclamations. He turned to *Merriam-Webster's Collegiate Dictionary* for a definition of "fitness" and being "fit"; it read, "the ability to transmit genes and being healthy." Glassman did not think that was a good definition. So he looked through exercise science sources and claimed, "the National Strength and Conditioning Association (NSCA), the most respected publisher in exercise physiology, in its highly authoritative 'Essentials of Strength and Conditioning,' does not even attempt a definition."[10] How can scientists who study fitness not have a definition, Glassman wondered. What were they studying? What were they measuring? As the son of a "rocket scientist" with a doctorate in "Scientific Systems," this made no sense to Glassman; it was not scientific. You cannot measure something that you do not define. So, he and CrossFit came up with a definition that was contrarian (no surprise) at the time because it did not focus on endurance but included elements of power, strength, and diet.

CrossFit defines fitness in a few ways. The first is like a Physics 101 definition: "work capacity over broad time and modal domains." (Physicists would say "work over modal domains" to be more precise because "work capacity" is not a physics concept and "work" implies "over time.") Work capacity over broad time and modal domains is simple: How many miles can you run if I say to run for twenty minutes (WOD One)? Or, if I say to squat one hundred pounds, how many times can you do it in five minutes (WOD Two)? Maybe put those two together and say, how many miles and one-hundred-pound squats can you do in thirty minutes if you run a mile and then do ten squats for as many rounds as possible (WOD Three)? This is work capacity (number of miles and hundred-pound squats) over broad time (five, twenty, or thirty minutes) and modal domains (squatting, running, doing both together).

What CrossFit claims to do, however, is not just to observe work capacity but to *increase* work capacity. The hypothesis is that CrossFit increases work capacity over broad time and modal domains. Experiments can be performed to assess this increased work capacity: perform all these workouts on the first three days of January, do CrossFit for six months, and then perform better on these WODs when done again on the first three days in June. If one does more of everything, then CrossFit has *increased work capacity across broad time and modal domains; CrossFit has made someone fitter*. Doing CrossFit definitely makes someone better at CrossFit.

In a video posted to the *CrossFit Journal* webpage titled "Defining CrossFit," Glassman is instructing a group of coaches on this definition. He says, "CrossFit is the application of the fundamentals of Newtonian mechanics to human movement," and people are nodding enthusiastically.[11] A consultation with a physicist reveals that this is a somewhat silly thing to say as everything that happens on Earth is the application of Newtonian mechanics: a human sitting in a chair, a laptop sitting on a desk, a dog chasing a ball, and the apple falling from the tree are all applications of Newtonian mechanics.[12] Newtonian mechanics is a mathematical representation of the physical world; if something exists in the universe, the laws of Newtonian mechanics apply. But the turn of phrase is an excellent marketing strategy to leverage scientific authority if the audience does not know that saying "the application of Newtonian mechanics" is, while accurate, not unique to CrossFit (and could also be used to describe them sitting and listening to the lecture).

In another video, titled "Real Science," Glassman is once again lecturing to an audience and talking about how no one has critiqued his definitions of fitness:

> I haven't found any rational, logical, scientific nor intelligent criticism of what we're doing, which is just amazing to me. . . . No one's taken on "work capacity across broad time and modal domains" or evidence-based fitness [which is] that we want measurables or repeatable data, regarding

power output or the fundamentals of kinematics that apply to all things that move everywhere in the universe also need to be applied to looking at human performance. You know, we—we're not challenged on that front. And so we remain on the technical front, on the scientific level entirely, entirely unimpeded. And when you run what we're doing by an engineer, by a physicist, by a mathematician, by a chemist, they're like, "Of course that's what you're doing." I mean, they fully get it. Not only does it make sense, but they can't imagine another way to look at human performance.

We've insulated ourselves from reproach, from those that know science and know it well. [What we're doing is] measurable. You can graph it. We're doing real science here.[13]

At the bottom of the "Defining CrossFit" video, there are eighty-one comments, many of them extensive about how imprecise and subjective the definition of "work capacity across broad time and modal domains" is. For example, Paul writes (edited for length),

The definition that CrossFit chooses is so broad and inclusive virtually anything could qualify.

Constantly Varied: subjective. CrossFit varies lots of movements, but far from everything it could.

Functional: subjective. [How is a handstand walk functional?]

High Intensity: subjective. Is a Marathon high intensity? 7 day hike/climb/bike? 1RM squat? Is a 12 second 100m dash intense for Usain Bolt? You?

Is CrossFit truly Varied? I've seen Fran come up a few times, yet have never seen basic things like any sort of throwing (Ok wall balls, but not Shot put, javelin, baseball) or any real sport WOD (i.e., Basketball, Soccer, swimming, skiing, hockey . . .) Many things are excluded but not by definition. I presume they are excluded out of practicality. Is the Hopper supposed to be practical too? Or is everything really in there it just hasn't come out yet? I know smashing a pole into the ground with a sledgehammer was so maybe I should have more faith.

All to say, it's all up for interpretation.

And show some math instead of just hiding behind an aura of science, which you are quick to criticize (i.e., Peer Reviewed, yes, I know the faults

> but you are not Copernicus). I have yet to see any experiment closely approximating a randomized control trial show any meaningful conclusions about CrossFit. "CrossFit makes you better at CrossFit!?" No way!
>
> Also, why do you pretend CrossFit is about Newtonian physics? If a 200lb athlete runs a 20min 5K run and a 110lb athlete runs it in 19minutes59 seconds who won the race? The larger athlete did more work but the lighter athlete was faster. Not to mention not a single post of performance is in ft lbs/sec. You didn't convert it for the Games to determine a winner.[14]

Paul has two main arguments with the "scientific" nature of CrossFit's definitions. First, the definition is too imprecise. Anything and everything could be considered CrossFit, yet not everything is included. Therefore, it is up for interpretation. "Natural science" is not up for interpretation; Aristotelian philosophy of nature is. Second, Paul wonders about the actual measurement of physical quantities. Paul gives the example of the 200-pound athlete versus the 110-pound athlete: if work capacity is the definition of fitness, the weight of the individuals would be considered when deciding who did more work, CrossFit's definition. But even in the CrossFit Games, actual work is not assessed to determine the fittest man or woman on Earth, just who finished first or did more repetitions. Therefore, CrossFit uses an indirect measure of work by assessing time, which, technically, is not the direct application of physics. If one wanted to measure the physical quantity of "work," one would need to measure it in joules, a unit of energy, and it would take an instrument that measures joules. If you do not measure joules, you are not measuring work or even "work capacity."

The linguistic focus on "work capacity" and "increased work capacity" in the CrossFit definition of fitness is meant to seem empirically driven; they can be tested: Can you do CrossFit workouts faster today than yesterday? However, as Paul notes, there is some fuzziness to this definition, allowing for significant subjectivity and interpretation.

In another example in the video for "Defining CrossFit," an audience member of the lecture poses a question (the question is unclear in the video), and Glassman wavers on his commitment to science and answers the man's question with,

I'm a math guy. Science doesn't prove; math proves. What science does is it will give, [he begins counting on his fingers] we have conjecture, we have hypothesis, we have theory, and we have law. Proof is involved in none of those four pieces [of science].

This isn't my first rodeo. . . . Yeah, we're on solid, solid scientific ground, and I enjoy this kind of interaction [i.e., debate about science]. But we've [CrossFit] got our ducks in a row, and we've got a science team. I got scientists behind me that are world-class, PhD physicists, PhD mathematicians, PhD electrical engineers, rocket scientists, people that have published extensively on science and the scientific method.[15]

In this videoed interaction at a coaching course where Glassman is lecturing, Glassman is challenged on the scientific aspects of CrossFit (he does not respond to Paul in the comments section of the video). In his response, first he says that he prefers to align CrossFit with math rather than science. "Science doesn't prove; math proves." But then he says, "We're on solid, solid scientific ground" with "ducks in a row" with a world-class "science team." He is aiming to accomplish two goals in this equivocation and proclamation. His equivocation is in reaction to some members of the audience of the video challenging his use of science. So, he throws science under the bus: it does not "prove"; math does. His claim that he is a "math guy" "counting things" aims to do what Merry argues counting things does, giving an aura of objectivity. But what Glassman decides to count is interpretive rather than objective: thrusters and T2B instead of a heart rate or the volume of sweat in a wrung-out postworkout T-shirt. He enumerates one thing (over others) and then tallies those things; this is auditing. Yet his return to claiming that science supports the CrossFit approach at the end of his remarks reflects an effort to legitimize what CrossFit is doing because science has long held a prestige position in society, an arbiter of expertise and authority. He wants to be doing science because science legitimates what he is doing as "better" according to the value structures of expertise. CrossFit tries to appear more scientific by using numbers and rankings, which really is a form of accounting, "scientific management," or audit culture.

CrossFit's second fitness definition defines three "fitness standards," which are outlined in a *CrossFit Journal* paper titled "What Is Fitness?" The first fitness standard is the *ability* to perform all these skills:

1. Cardiovascular/respiratory endurance—The ability of body systems to gather, process and deliver oxygen.
2. Stamina—The ability of body systems to process, deliver, store and utilize energy.
3. Strength—The ability of a muscular unit, or combination of muscular units, to apply force.
4. Flexibility—The ability to maximize the range of motion at a given joint.
5. Power—The ability of a muscular unit, or combination of muscular units, to apply maximum force in minimum time.
6. Speed—The ability to minimize the time cycle of a repeated movement.
7. Coordination—The ability to combine several distinct movement patterns into a singular distinct movement.
8. Agility—The ability to minimize transition time from one movement pattern to another.
9. Balance—The ability to control the placement of the body's center of gravity in relation to its support base.
10. Accuracy—The ability to control movement in a given direction or at a given intensity.[16]

In other words, someone is fit if one is *capable* in each of these skills. Sure, a triathlete is overly capable in the first, but can she produce power, does she have coordination, and is she accurate? Someone who claims to be fit or is identified as "the fittest on Earth" *should* be capable in each of these.

The second fitness standard according to this *CrossFit Journal* article is about *rank* in these abilities: "Picture a hopper loaded with an infinite number of physical challenges where no selective mechanism is operative and being asked to perform feats randomly drawn from the hopper. This model suggests that your fitness can be measured by your capacity to perform well at these tasks in *relation to other individuals*."[17] Fitness *should* be about performing physical tasks better than others.

Finally, the third fitness standard is to be capable in the three human metabolic pathways—oxidative, glycolytic, and phosphagen—that provide energy for human action. The oxidative is the most well-known pathway: cardiovascular exercises use oxygen to fuel the work performed. This is the exercise in which you can talk while you do it. Glycolytic uses glycogen in the muscles, and this is the exercise in which you cannot talk while you do it because you are breathing too hard. Lastly, the phosphagen pathway is about pure power production, which lasts less than ten seconds and uses cellular power (ATP). According to CrossFit, fitness *should* be defined based on one's ability to tap into these various systems effectively to produce work, to be coordinated as well as fast and have stamina, and to be better in all these areas than other people.

If you run what CrossFit is doing by those who study the enumeration of everyday tasks or the quantification of aspects of life, they would say that this is auditing, applying the standards of accounting to nonfinancial areas of social life; they might even call it what Frederick Taylor did in 1913: scientific management. But it is not science. It is defining something, creating a scoring system based on that definition, and then assessing a target (fitness standards) on the basis of that scoring system. The numbers seem to be "neutral" and to be governed by math. But CrossFit's definitions and standards hark back to systems developed by West Point, Frederick Taylor, and Henry Ford, which began the enumeration of activities and the accumulation of those numbers into a score or grade to reward people with the highest marks. This was not about science or math but about improving labor productivity and thus a company's bottom line; it is neoliberal capitalism. CrossFit is an audit system. CrossFit gyms embrace an audit culture in which standards defined by CrossFit HQ are monitored. CrossFitters have auditing subjectivities because they internalize and police these standards to know if they are exercising right.[18]

The third and final definition of CrossFit is "CrossFit in 100 Words," or,

Eat meat and vegetables, nuts and seeds, some fruit, little starch and no sugar. Keep intake to levels that will support exercise but not body fat.

Practice and train major lifts: deadlift, clean, squat, presses, clean-and-jerk, and snatch. Similarly, master the basics of gymnastics: pull-ups, dips, rope climb, push-ups, sit-ups, presses to handstand, pirouettes, flips, splits, and holds. Bike, run, swim, row, etc. hard and fast.

Five or six days per week, mix these elements in as many combinations and patterns as creativity will allow. Routine is the enemy. Keep workouts short and intense.

Regularly learn and play new sport.[19]

The hundred-word definition reads more like a philosophy of fitness or religious commandments: what to eat (meat and veggies), what not to eat (sugar or too much starch), what to do (deadlift, press, handstands, etc.), how to do it (hard and fast), when to do it (five or six times a week), what not to do (follow a routine), and even more general adages such as "learn" and "play." This "definition" is more aligned with philosophy than with physics.

In fact, there were comments alongside Paul's earlier comment that disagreed with Glassman's premise that CrossFit is based on science, and still others argued that it did not matter even if it was not. For example, Cam writes, "CrossFit is a PHILOSOPHY of training towards higher work capacity across broad time and modal domains. It is NOT a training system as it is not even close to being clearly defined in terms of frequency, intensity, or volume (so we can get rid of the "functional movements" and "high intensity" jargon)."[20] Meanwhile, Thomas does not think CrossFit's greatest contribution has anything to do with science or philosophy; he writes,

> CrossFit's greatest contribution is not the definition of fitness, but rather the level of community the program builds. I have never seen a single CrossFitter concerned with actually measuring their work capacity across broad time and modal domains. Yes, they care about their level of fitness, but not to the degree that is defined by HQ. The idea of plotting a graph of their fitness or trying to estimate their ability in the 10 skills is nebulous and mostly useless for an individual person. The true power of the program is its ability to bring people together, build community, and motivate each other through a workout.[21]

Yes, CrossFit *feels* like science, with its definition, its enumeration, and its plotting of those numbers onto a graph or into a notebook to illustrate improvement. It can even be identified as "scientific management." But there are serious holes in its logic, as pointed out in internet-style peer review. If we use the definition of "audit," we see that CrossFit "science" is not the kind used in the laboratory but in the cubicle to improve worker productivity. There is a moral undergirding of the prescriptive nature of CrossFit. It does not just observe what one does or what one eats but rather prescribes how to do something (sixty-five pounds on the barbell for thrusters or as "Rx'ed") and how to eat. Strathern notes that in audit culture, a good measure of something ceases to be a good measure when there is a target to achieve. When a target is part of the equation, the math takes on moral weight. With auditing measurements came a new morality of attainment, or the concept of improvement. Improvement is about effort and results, not about what is. It is the addition of "increased" in the "work capacity" definition that locates CrossFit in the moral world of audit culture, with a search for a by-the-numbers-better-than-yesterday self.

CrossFit's "Evolutionary Science"

In addition to math, CrossFit likes to tap into scientific frameworks around evolution. Now, instead of focusing on numbers, CrossFitters are supposed to focus on "functional" exercises, those that are required "by life" and are essential to live independently. In a whiteboard animation video on the CrossFit website defining functional movement, a male voice narrates the following while an illustrating hand draws:

> Functional movements are what prepared you for life: squatting, running, jumping, throwing, pulling, picking things up—all predate gyms by thousands of years [drawings of a woman running, a man in a suit and tie with a briefcase jumping over a puddle, and a man in an animal hide holding a large stone over his head when the voice says 'thousands of years']. They weren't invented by anyone, and they're found everywhere. They are what our bodies were meant to do. It's in our DNA. CrossFit workouts use functional movements because they are so much more effective for life outside the gym.[22]

CrossFit movements are human movements, in our DNA, part of our evolutionary trajectory. CrossFit taps into evolutionary science to make claims about its effectiveness as a fitness regimen evinced in the function of the movements.

Humans can do many movements, but we are uniquely adapted to walk upright for a long period of time. But we also have the capacity to perform short spurts of high-power movements, like sprinting or jumping. One of the movements that humans' ape ancestors evolved to perform, which we benefit from but do not make use of in our everyday lives, is swinging from tree branch to tree branch. We have thumbs uniquely forged to grip things, and our shoulder joints allow us to move our arms in an entire circle. Because of these unique attributes, humans have retained the ability to brachiate, or the locomotor capacity to swing through the trees. This is also the movement of the front crawl or backstroke in swimming. All living apes have the anatomy to do this. We do not usually move like this. (When was the last time you swung between trees, let alone across "the monkey bars"—a misnomer because monkeys, unlike apes, cannot brachiate—at the local park's jungle gym?) But we can. It is in our DNA.

According to CrossFit, "functional" fitness seems like an easily defined thing—a movement that we were born to do, that is in our DNA, that was not invented but just existed. Upon closer inspection, though, it taps into not only unique movements that we have evolved to perform but also those found useful during extreme situations like war. Perhaps, like the use of physics discussed earlier, this is a clever way to tap into evolutionary science to make claims about the utility and supremacy of the CrossFit method. There is a significant desire to tap into ancestral ways of life to lend credibility to the regimen, as when Glassman declared on *60 Minutes* that he "delivered" to people their genetic potential as he pointed to a woman doing a workout: "Look at her. She was meant to look like that. That's what nature would have carved from her a million years ago. Or she'd have been eaten." Here CrossFit is tapping into evolutionary science to validate its regimen, even if some of that evolutionary "science" is not accurate. Humans were not around a million years ago.

In addition to functional movements, CrossFit found common ground with the "paleo" diet. The first-ever CrossFit affiliate was founded in Seattle, and one of those new affiliate owners was a man named Robb Wolf. Wolf is a biochemist and powerlifter who wrote a book called *The Paleo Solution: The Original Human Diet*, which, according to the website, claims that "The Paleo diet is the healthiest way you can eat because it is the ONLY nutritional approach that works with your genetics to help you stay lean, strong and energetic!"[23]

As mentioned earlier, during my research, when people learned that I was an anthropologist, they all wanted to know if I did "paleo," which

I had not heard of before my research on CrossFit. When I said no, they lectured me on the evolutionary basis of the diet. According to Wolf and many of the CrossFitters I encountered, the paleo diet is grounded in evolutionary theory. I had not heard of this diet in my anthropology courses or in the twenty years of anthropological study I had conducted before I entered a CrossFit gym. I had taken many biological anthropology courses, and not once did any faculty member claim that there was one healthy way to eat across all of human existence. In fact, Herman Pontzer, a premier evolutionary anthropologist who studies metabolic adaptations and has lived with the Hadza, hunters and gatherers in Tanzania, affirms, "There's a lot of cherry-picking of the evidence that's out there to suggest that all hunter-gatherer diets or past ancestral diets were carnivore-like, with a lot of meat and hardly any fruits and vegetables, and there's just absolutely no evidence for that at all. The reality is that people ate and still do eat a wide variety of diets."[24] In a magazine article for *American Scientist*, Pontzer is quoted as saying, "Traditional foraging adaptations are diverse. Although some traditional societies (Arctic communities, for example) do tend to rely on meat, many others (including equatorial ones) do not." His research on diet and foraging strategies among the Hadza shows that meat has provided a relatively small proportion of the calories in their diet. "Like the people in many other traditional societies, they consume large amount of carbohydrates, berries, fiber, and honey."[25]

Anthropologists examine the diets of contemporary humans living a hunting and gathering lifestyle (such as the Hadza) and those of archaic humans who have now gone extinct (*Homo erectus* and *Homo neanderthalensis*) to understand how humans have evolved, including what they have evolved to eat. Briana Pobiner, a research scientist at the Smithsonian's National Museum of Natural History, wrote an article about the various ways anthropologists examine fossils to try to figure out the diets of early humans and our nonhuman ancestors. Anthropologists examine skeletal morphology, or the size and shape of early human skulls and teeth, which can tell us something about chewing muscle and strength. They also examine dental microwear to see what the individual was eating, especially in the final weeks of their life. If there are tiny pits, then it was probably seeds or nuts; if striations are visible, then it was probably grass, leaves, or flesh. Anthropologists also examine remnants of plants in the fossil record using carbon isotopes. Different plants leave different carbon isotope compositions, which can offer a general understanding of the kinds of plants that were available at a given time and thus what the early humans ate. Finally, plant microfossils, usually starch grains or silica, can be found in mouths of early human fossils. Pobiner argues that "using different lines of evidence, paleoanthropologists can work toward seemingly lofty goals like estimating the proportion of different kinds of foods like plants, meat, and insects in prehistoric diets."[26]

Many people believe that Neanderthals (*Homo neanderthalensis*), or what is commonly meant when someone says "caveman," such as the one drawn in the CrossFit functional fitness whiteboard animation, ate mostly protein. The biological anthropologists Cara Ocobock, Sara Lacy, and Alexandra Niclou argue that "we now recognize that Neanderthal diets varied seasonally and geographically" and included date palms and grass seeds (Southwest Asia), herbaceous plants and grass seeds (Eastern Mediterranean), marine mammals (Western Mediterranean), shellfish, mosses, and mushrooms (Southern Atlantic Coast), and large terrestrial mammals and cooked starches (Northern Atlantic Coast).[27] In a paper in the *Proceedings of the National Academy of Sciences*, paleoanthropologists write that despite the widely accepted idea that prehistoric diets included an increase in animal tissue over time as our prehistoric ancestors became more human, there is no evidence for this between 2.6 and 1.2 million years ago. In other words, beginning with *Homo erectus*, it seems that our ancestors did not eat more meat than those before *Homo erectus*, suggesting that what makes humans human is not based on eating more meat.[28]

There is considerable scientific research on the diets of contemporary hunters and gatherers, nonhuman ancestors, and early and extinct humans, including the "caveman" or Neanderthal. None of this research supports Robb Wolf's claim that the "paleo diet," which is largely based on protein consumption, was in fact the "original human diet based on genetics." Indeed, Wolf's claim is confusing for someone studying Neanderthal diets because there is no such thing as an "original human diet." Humans have been eating lots of carbs (and seeds and flesh) for much of nonhuman (hominin) and human (*Homo sapiens*) history. Even "caveman" diets included a lot more cooked starches than what is commonly thought.

In other words, evolutionary science does not support the evolutionary claims made by CrossFit. Humans are what biological anthropologists call "generalists"; there is no one human diet. CrossFit is not based on evolutionary science. It just likes to say it is.

What is sitting in the room with this theory of evolutionary science at CrossFit as an underlying code are the tropes of heroes we discussed earlier. The idea of a "fittest" person is an afterlife of evolutionary notions of "survival of the fittest," a phase coined by Herbert Spencer in his reading of Darwin's *Origins of Species*. Spencer wore many hats, one of them as an "armchair" anthropologist, conjecturing theories of linear human social evolution by reading the journals of explorers and missionaries from the "comfort of his armchair." He wrote prolifically during the nineteenth century, as the American West was being "won" and Indigenous people in the Americas were being slaughtered, often with the argument that their technology was not as "advanced" as that of the white missionaries and frontiersmen. This notion of "winning" was linked to the notion of the "survival of the fittest."

This phrase and theory have been the foundation of white supremacist conceptualizations of human biological and social evolution through the eugenics movement. According to the movement's founder, Francis Dalton, eugenics "is the science which deals with all influences that improve the inborn qualities of a race; also, with those that develop them to the utmost advantage."[29] In more colloquial terms, eugenics is the pseudoscientific study of the inherent superiority of white people and the methods and practices by which to keep them superior. These have included marriage laws and sterilization policies targeting nonwhite populations to keep the white gene pool "pure."

Through the mapping of the human genome, it has been revealed that race is not mapped onto genes and that there is no scientific justification for racial groups, let alone racial hierarchies. Nonetheless, eugenics is still popular in certain pockets of the US and is used to support ideologies of white supremacy and practices of racial violence against nonwhite people. It is on this backdrop that Musselman writes that the CrossFit Games has undertones of social Darwinism: the idea of there being a "fittest" person, that he or she is crowned because they "survived" harrowing physical and mental tests, that all of these are white men and women, and that these abilities are inherent or genetic, all of which are afterlives of eugenics arguments that white people are a "scientifically-supported" "superior race."[30] According to anthropologists, this is absolutely not true.

CrossFit's Vigilante Science

As we saw earlier, when Glassman looked for definitions of "fitness" and found none by the National Strength and Conditioning Association, he had CrossFit create its own. He argued that he was the first to adequately define "fitness" and then set up a way to measure it. He has also claimed that while sometimes people attack him on personal grounds, he has not "found any rational, logical, scientific nor intelligent criticism" of what CrossFit is doing.[31] Instead, he has found problems with the fitness industry's scientific claims. This stance is nowhere more obvious than in his critique of the *Journal of Strength and Conditioning Research*, which published an article that claimed that CrossFit increased maximal aerobic fitness and body composition but that it also had high injury rates.

The research was done by the Ohio State University's kinesiology department using members of a local CrossFit affiliate. After the paper was published, CrossFit did not believe the injury rate data. Russell Berger, a known enforcer of CrossFit ideals, veteran Army Ranger, and Glassman's bodyguard, called the local CrossFit affiliate associated with the research. The owner gave Berger the names of those who were involved in the study (despite their having been offered anonymity or recorded as simply a number by the researchers). Berger then called some of the CrossFit members involved, and "they all confirmed that they were not injured but had failed to show up to the final test due to lack of time or interest."[32]

After a member of the CrossFit gym who worked as a clinical researcher and served as the volunteer study coordinator for the Ohio State researchers questioned the "validity of the research" on the basis of follow-up protocols and the claims that these participants made to Berger on the phone about not being injured, CrossFit dug deeper into the study, trying to reveal its lack of scientific rigor.[33] They found that the study did not have IRB (Institutional Review Board) approval, which is an ethical approval required for research with humans. It was also revealed that during the peer-review process, the editor of the journal required information on injury rates for the article to be approved for publication by the journal. CrossFit thus proposed that the researchers made up the injury rates, attributing injury to those who failed to show up for the final test. The Ohio State professor resigned, the journal corrected and then retracted the article, and several lawsuits were filed. Ohio State settled with the CrossFit gym owner. A federal judge in California found that the NSCA acted in bad faith when withholding documents and lying under oath and ordered it to pay CrossFit's legal fees and undisclosed damages.[34] Most importantly, CrossFit claimed that university kinesiology departments were not doing sound research. Glassman and CrossFit also dug deeper into the NCSA.

Glassman found that funding for the NCSA and many fitness and nutrition research projects across the US university landscape were partially funded by PepsiCo. A deep dive into the sugar industry revealed that it was funding research on strength and conditioning organizations, health nonprofits, diabetes foundations, and foundations supporting the Centers for Disease Control (CDC) and National Institutes of Health (NIH). A 2016 Boston University study found that Coca-Cola and PepsiCo funded ninety-six national health and medical groups.[35] This information was used by CrossFit to vindicate Glassman and CrossFit's claims that the NCSA was involved in corrupt practices and shoddy science. Glassman declared war on Big Soda; he hired a lobbying group and went to Washington, DC, with his bodyguards to see what he could do about the influence of the sugar industry.[36] It was unconscionable, Glassman claimed, that Big Soda, which is partially to blame for many chronic disease problems facing Americans, was waist deep in funding the science that supported claims that exercise was more important than nutrition for health markers. In other words, the science that Coca-Cola and PepsiCo funded skipped over "don't drink caloric-dense soft drinks" recommendations and concluded with "just get enough exercise." In 2018, Michael Easter reported that Glassman was taking on health care by creating CrossFit Health and a training course for physicians because their medical school training was negligent on nutrition and exercise information but full of pharmacology.[37] Glassman, a proud college dropout, was declaring that his scientific method was sounder than that of universities and national associations that published scientific journals. He mobilized his fitness empire to rectify this injustice by schooling physicians and laypeople on the benefits of his "scientifically sound" CrossFit method. CrossFit was the vigilante science in town, righteously taking on the corrupt government and officials (the "law") and protecting Americans—despite, as we have seen, the method actually being audit based and not scientifically or mathematically based.

The History and Value of Science

Western science is not just about key figures, such as Bacon or Aristotle, who through noble pursuits find the natural laws of the universe. Rather, there is a complex history of power and legitimacy that undergirds definitions of science and scientific knowledge. Modern Western science became the dominant method of thought and inquiry not because it was better than other methods or because European scientists were the first to "discover" things but rather because modern Western science colonized other forms of scientific inquiry through Christian imperialism. The new ideas of Francis Bacon (and others) during the 1600s found their way to colonies, were implemented in colonized educational systems, and were used to legitimate Christian, European dominance.[38] Science is never outside of the systems—of power and value—that produce it, despite its claim in finding natural, objective law. Bruno Latour, a renowned philosopher of science, claims that scientific literature, laboratory activities, institutional contexts that fund or support science, and the ways in which discoveries or inventions occur are all fundamentally shaped by social contexts, political power, and ideological constructs.[39]

Brian Pronger examines the contexts and power that undergird the fitness industry. He argues that the "technology of physical fitness" is composed of texts, practices, and procedures that produce human life in controlled ways. These texts include popular images in magazines, film, television, and social media that reproduce understandings of a "fit" body: lean, muscular, and young. The sociocultural practices include governmental policies and initiatives of physical fitness, including college degrees in kinesiology, definitions created by national associations, local community centers with diet and fitness programs or youth sports initiatives such as the "President's Physical Fitness Tests" that Eisenhower established but Reagan epitomized, and the multitrillion-dollar fitness industry. Body procedures include actual fitness regimens like CrossFit: how to eat, what to lift, how fast to go, when to stop, who to do this with, and so on. What this entire "discursive system" produces, according to Pronger, is a particular way of being, one that locates physical fitness in rigid technological definitions rather than in the love, joy, or pleasure of movement. He calls this "body fascism."[40] Another way to think of this can be linked back to the walk: Did you get your ten thousand steps in, or did you enjoy your afternoon walk? The current state of physical fitness is to "count" the steps, not the pleasure.

The anthropologist Hugh Gusterson argues that science—I am including exercise science here—has been thought to somehow live outside of culture, unlike other systems of knowledge production, such as shamanism. This is because of the ideological power of science and scientific discourses in Western society, often forged through "antagonistic struggles between rival networks of scientists." The anthropology of science investigates how these factions of science "remake society as [scientists] go about their scientific work."[41] Scientists and ideologies of science (for example, inductive versus deductive methods, eugenics versus contemporary paleoanthropology) exercise considerable power in society due to their location in prestige institutions (universities, laboratories, national associations) and with people holding advanced degrees from these prestige institutions (PhDs and "rocket scientists"). But as we have seen, science is also appropriated (by PepsiCo, Robb Wolf and the diet book industry), contested (Ohio State versus CrossFit), and undermined (auditing being mistaken for science) with claims from various social groups.

CrossFit took its "solid scientific foundation" and the ruthless ferocity of Glassman and other members of CrossFit HQ and went after the "corrupt" academic research industry. The company created sections of CrossFit, such as CrossFit Health, to address this "corruption" and "failure" by governmental institutions, thus swooping in like vigilante superheroes to provide their own—better, more scientific, less corrupted by Big Soda—version. They—CrossFit and Glassman—would save the scientific and health day! Even if their scientific claims were not entirely true. They would take on the corrupt enemy—the government, the lobbyist, corporate America, academia, scholarship—through their fitness methodology, gyms, community, website, the *CrossFit Journal* and by using pithy maxims on Twitter (now known as X). This all came to a head in 2020 when the end times seemed upon us.

7

This Was Not the Apocalypse We Trained For!

The history of religion (and particularly American religion, with its sectarian impulse) teaches us that conditions for schism develop after the unifying enthusiasm of the founding-era subsides and debates over community consensus around moral action, doctrine, or communal boundaries arise.
—Cody Musselman, "Survival of the CrossFittest"

I walk into the gym halfway through the marathon row. Eight men, from their late twenties to early fifties, are lined up and rowing on stationary rowing machines called "ergs." They all have pools of sweat on the floor beneath them, and they are drenched. I knew they were planning on doing this. Coach Peter had decided last minute to organize a "marathon row" and alerted me to the workout. Maybe I would find it interesting, or did I want to do it? I'm five feet two inches tall; the last workout I want to do is row forty-two thousand meters on an erg.

I walk over and check their progress. The erg has a screen that displays various units—watts, time, average five-hundred-meter split, and so on; I could see how far they had rowed already. When I arrive, they have been rowing for ninety minutes straight. No wonder they are drenched. Coach Peter, a tall white guy who had been an elite rower at one time in his life, is rowing with one hand as he holds a banana in his other. He uses his teeth to peel it open and begins eating it while still rowing. "You can still join us," he tells me. I laugh and say, "I'm going to simply observe this one. Why did you do this, set this up at the last minute? Why didn't you train for it, like one would a running marathon?" He does not stop rowing or eating his banana; his legs and arms are cramping, so he must get some potassium into his system, he tells me. He takes a big bite and with a mouth full of banana says, "Because you never know when shit is going to hit the fan. I want to show these guys our training in the gym prepares us to do something like this at the last minute."

I let his words sink in as I look at the other rowers. I know one is a corporate lawyer and another is a stock trader in Asian markets. I am not sure what the other men do for a living, but they are all professionals, white-collar, type-A types. I wonder, When will these men ever have to row a marathon at a moment's notice? Are there boats on the East River or other Brooklyn waterways that might have standing canoes or kayaks when "shit hits the fan" and we need to escape a burning, exploding city? I am American; I have been thoroughly inundated with every kind of apocalyptic image. Will these kinds of people—white, male, elite—not be at the top of the list for rescue or safe hiding when the apocalypse comes? But this is just it; these men would not have to wait to be rescued; they could take their survival into their own hands, hero style, and Coach Peter is illustrating this in today's row. It is not *despite* the last-minute decision to do it, the pools of sweat generated, the cramping in their body from their efforts, and the three hours it would take them to finish that these men would do this rowing workout; it is *because* of it. Cramps, dehydration, and severe fatigue are not enough to stop them from finishing today. And these symptoms would not prohibit them from doing such a wild and crazy physical task if ever the real world demanded it. They are heroes, ready today and when shit hits the fan.

All of them finished the marathon row. I saw a few of them later in the week and asked how they felt. They replied in both physical and mental terms. "My body held up better than I thought. I'm surprised! Now I know I can do something like that if I ever needed to," a fifty-one-year old told me. In the United States, "shit hitting the fan" can be a reference to the end times; in my local CrossFit gym, it was often used this way. And Coach Peter and his participants were ready for it.

In my Goth-style Brooklyn gym, I heard a lot about the zombie apocalypse: who was going to survive it, whom people wanted on their "team" when it happened, and what people were doing to train for it. The tongue-in-cheek statements about a zombie apocalypse came mostly from nonevangelicals or nonmilitary CrossFitters. Without getting into the weeds, the zombie is not a neutral being.[1] It, like the US military, has roots and ties to US imperialism, colonial and capitalist domination, and racial inequalities. Therefore, not only do Hero and Girl workouts remind people of the relationship between CrossFit and disaster, war, and death—especially the Hero WODs—but everyday CrossFit workouts are laced with disaster or war preparedness and fears of upended worlds from nonwhite Others. In another gym across the country, deep in a religious, red state, a CrossFit gym had a giant image on the wall. It is a white, blond man with a CrossFit T-shirt on and black sunglasses. He is pointing up and has his mouth open; it looks like he is at the CrossFit Games, and he is shouting to the crowd, to which he is pointing. On this image is a quotation: "Train hard, train smart, train to survive." This image also links this CrossFit gym's training with surviving, perhaps, as Glassman says in his *60 Minutes* interview, for war, for mugging, or for a cancer diagnosis. The end is coming. Are you prepared? CrossFit will prepare you.

American Apocalypse

Narratives of the end times are everywhere in contemporary American popular culture. There are television shows (*The Walking Dead*), films (*Day after Tomorrow, Independence Day*, many recent superhero movies), comic books (superhero ones), young-adult fiction (the *Left Behind* series), adult fiction (Margaret Atwood's *MaddAddam* trilogy), and so on; even the United States' Centers for Disease Control had a zombie apocalypse preparedness webpage, which included lesson plans for middle-school-aged children in 2019.[2] But these speculative fiction or religious-based stories about the end times are not new; American culture has always been apocalyptic.[3]

The New England Puritans and pilgrims hoped to establish the book of Revelation's "New Jerusalem," and early American Christians were asked to look out for signs of the imminent "Second Coming" of Christ. There were a couple of "Great Awakenings," the Second drawing huge crowds with emotional appeals to convert before the imminent Second Coming. Christian sects splintered off with new American versions of the return of Christ, including the United Society of Believers in Christ's Second Appearing (also known as the Shakers), the Church of Jesus Christ of Latter-day Saints (also known as Mormons), and those who followed William Miller and his Millerism (who today are known as the Jehovah's Witnesses and the Seventh-day Adventists). Soon millennialism and apocalypticism moved from church pulpits and pews to American culture more broadly, including in battle hymns, literature, and poetry and on to present-day film, television, games, music, and CDC recommendations for preparing children for disaster. In other words, even though apocalyptic fever seems to be everywhere right now—pandemics, zombies, aliens, artificial intelligence, melting ice caps, plagues, and so on—American culture has always been apocalyptic.[4]

What is the apocalypse? The term has Greek origins and means "to uncover, unveil, or reveal."[5] Apocalypse is the revealing of ultimate truths at the end times. In Christianity, this *revelation* is unveiled in biblical prophecy. There are two main perspectives about the biblical end times: postmillennialism and premillennialism.[6] In the historian Matthew Sutton's book *American Apocalypse*, he examines how in the mid-1800s, many white American Christians felt optimistic about the future and longed for the "millennium" or a thousand-year period "of peace, prosperity, and righteousness described in the book of Revelation, which [many American Protestants] hoped to help inaugurate through their own good works. They believed that the return of Christ would mark the conclusion of the millennium," hence the "post-" in "postmillennialism."[7] This apocalypse story was the most common in the United States for centuries. However, Sutton continues, following the French Revolution and its aftermath, many Protestant theologians in Europe were less optimistic about the future and felt that the apocalypse story needed revising.

In the latter half of the 1800s, the Irishman John Nelson Darby and his theological system called "dispensational premillennialism" argued that the Second Coming of Jesus was imminent and would include a "rapture."[8] The word "rapture" does not appear in the Bible, but it can be defined as "a dramatic experience in which all living Christians will mysteriously vanish from earth and the dead will rise to heaven." Those who are left behind would suffer a seven-year "tribulation" under a new leader, the Antichrist, who would be vanquished by Christ and his army of saints, "inaugurating Jesus's millennial reign on earth."[9] Premillennialism gained popularity in the United States in the 1860s–1870s as Darby toured the United States giving sermons. Although it is impossible to know how many American Christians embraced premillennialism, Sutton writes, "in the post–World War II era [there was a] tremendous surge in the number of evangelical churches that affirmed premillennialism."[10]

Sutton argues,

> Perceiving the United States as besieged by satanic forces—communism and secularism, family breakdown and government encroachment—Billy Sunday, Charles Fuller, Billy Graham, and many others took to the pulpit and airwaves to explain how biblical end-times prophecy made sense of a world ravaged by global wars, genocide, and the threat of nuclear extinction. Rather than withdraw from their communities to wait for Armageddon, they use what little time was left to warn of the coming Antichrist, save souls, and prepare the United States for God's final judgment. Their work helped define the major issues and controversies of the twentieth century, and they continue to exert a tremendous influence over the American mainstream today.[11]

Fears about the pending apocalypse did not stay in the evangelical Christian community alone. In the wake of this American Christian tradition, the notion of apocalypse moved from the pulpit to the cinema screen, bookstore, and internet. Sutton traces how apocalyptic ideas took hold everywhere, from the office of the US president to popular culture; due to cultural Christianity, "no part of American life [is] immune to Christian apocalypticism."[12] Even health and fitness regimens have been linked to preparation for the Second Coming, revealing in embodied form one's fitness for salvation when the time comes.[13] Sutton cites various Pew Research Center polls: a 2006 poll illustrates that 79 percent of Christians believe in the Second Coming, with 20 percent expecting it to happen in their lifetime; a 2010 poll reveals that "forty-one percent of all Americans (well over one hundred million people) and fifty-eight percent of white evangelicals believed that Jesus 'definitely' or 'probably' is going to return by 2050." Sutton claims that most of these believers may not understand the "complex theology" of apocalypse frameworks (premillennialism or postmillennialism), but the polls reveal "how widespread Christian apocalyptic ideas are and how thoroughly evangelical premillennialism has saturated American culture over the last one hundred and fifty years."[14] Americans live in the wake of "evangelicals' apocalyptic hopes, dreams, and nightmares," where apocalypticism is a "powerful lens through which to make sense of difficult or challenging eras." This "distinct form of Christian cultural engagement has impacted the world in profound ways."[15]

The apocalypse stories and their influence on cultural Christianity are highly racialized; most are grounded in white evangelical frameworks of the end times.[16] African American Christians were also influenced by premillennialism, but they followed the tradition of Black jeremiads against racial injustice. Black church "leaders longed for an end to inequality and anticipated the day when they would rule with Christ during the new millennium."[17] Prophecy was read in racialized ways in the United States, with African American Christians reading calls for equity and justice in the Bible while white American evangelical Christians generally did not.[18] Indigenous Americans experienced genocide and violence, their own apocalypse, during the takeover of their land by European intruders.[19] As a result, Indigenous versions of the end times include the decolonization of the present-day nation-state and a postapocalyptic/utopian world where the "Indians won."[20] Despite there being various versions of the apocalypse in American culture and literature, the one that has come to dominate is a white evangelical one.[21]

These Christian frameworks color "secular" understandings of the apocalypse. In 2018, I wrote a paper that examined how CrossFitters prepare for the "zombie apocalypse."[22] While I made the claim that the zombie, as a monster and as a bringer of the apocalypse made popular by the director George Romero, was secular, I have now come to see that any apocalypse—zombie or FBI raid at your compound—is an afterlife of Christianity. The rapture, violent Armageddon, and the apocalypse are all Christian notions, forged in churches, undergirded by Christian theology, disseminated from the pulpit or house church, and now, due to cultural Christianity, on our big and little screens, in novels, episodic shows, and films. The same apocalypse frameworks that shape mainstream Christian understandings of prophecy or cult charters and mass suicide events also emerge as afterlives in the preparing for the unknown unknown, the war on terror, the zombie apocalypse, or CrossFit ideology when "shit hits the fan."

Like other charismatic leaders during end-times scenarios, Greg Glassman tried to rally his followers during the COVID-19 pandemic. While there was an official line coming from CrossFit HQ to follow local governance orders, the "rabid libertarian" Glassman, with his history of fights against established authority and his deeply held belief that he is better at science than the scientists, called what the US government was doing "a failure." He thought his devotees would follow him in this fight. They did, until the beginning of June 2020, and then CrossFit itself began to crumble like the buildings in many apocalypse-based films.

In the United States, preparing for the end times is not a marginalized idea. It is everywhere, in our films, television shows, novels, young-adult literature, and fitness regimens. These versions of the end times are always violent. Preparing for a violent apocalypse using masculine, intense, varied, functional workouts, as CrossFit aims to train its adherents to do, fits into our national myths about the coming of the end of the world and the valor and heroic acts of a select few who could survive and protect their families and friends. But the apocalypse of the COVID-19 pandemic asked for care, quiet, staying at home, sitting on the couch, and letting the "real" heroes nurse the sick back to health.

This was not the apocalypse that CrossFitters had trained for.

2020

It all happened so fast—the fall of Greg Glassman and his version of CrossFit. It was June 2020, and I, like many people throughout the world, was in some sort of "lockdown" as the pandemic raged on. In the United States, the murder of George Floyd by police on May 25 in Minneapolis ruptured an already fragile country. The ripples of his cry "I can't breathe" as an officer kneeled on his neck were spreading to all corners of the nation, mobilizing massive street protests in almost every major and minor city. There were calls for criminal justice reform and shouts of "Black Lives Matter." George Floyd's murder and his cries that he could not breathe shook a nation three months into the respiratory-based pandemic.

Earlier, beginning in 2016, the same year CrossFit Games athletes were awarded a handgun as a prize and NBA superstars were calling for the end of gun violence, the football player Colin Kaepernick had kneeled during the national anthem at National Football League (NFL) games to protest police violence against his fellow Black Americans, but few people or organizations supported his choice. In 2018, Nike was one lone voice of support, following through on its contract with the quarterback and linking its "Just Do It" tagline with Kaepernick's "Know Your Rights." But Kaepernick had been blacklisted by NFL teams. By 2020, in the wake of Floyd's murder, even Roger Goodell, the commissioner of the NFL, was claiming that he was wrong in how he had handled Kaepernick's call for justice and that he and the NFL would do better to listen to Black players' voices.[23] The NFL was not alone. Companies were choosing a side, with most squarely landing on the side that claimed "Black Lives Matter" and making this statement publicly via black boxes on Twitter, Instagram, or Facebook, formal letters sent to emails via listservs, and posts on websites. George Floyd's murder had become a watershed moment in racial justice pursuits in the United States. Dual threats of pandemic and police violence were killing Americans, and it had to stop.

Unlike Goodell, Greg Glassman, the CEO and owner of CrossFit, made a very different choice. On June 3, Alyssa Royse, the owner of an affiliate in Seattle, now called Rocket Community Fitness but at the time called Rocket CrossFit, emailed the CrossFit CEO, Brian Mulvaney, to let him know that "Rocket" would probably be dropping its affiliation with the brand.[24] She wrote that the brand did not seem to share her values and that she had to keep telling people that her gym was not "that kind of CrossFit." She wrote that she loved CrossFit and had kept the name despite these cringeworthy moments—until COVID hit. She wrote a long email that CrossFit leadership had failed her and other affiliates: its "moral ambiguity" regarding the real deaths caused by COVID, especially in minority communities, and what she called the fat-shaming and racist posts (a "Fluffy Duck" post that I discuss shortly) that the social media accounts were sharing were the last straw. (Her entire email can be found on the Rocket Community Fitness website; it is about three thousand words and includes images of the social media posts she references.)[25] She implored CrossFit to do something, to say something about Black Lives Matter. She emphasized that silence was taking a stand. She concluded her "break up email" with, "We have been through so much together that it would simply be wrong to ghost you, even if it's just business. We all have decisions to make, and I trust that even if we do wind up doing it from different paths, we will still be making the world a better place. I will always wish we could do it together.

Love, Alyssa." Alyssa posted this previously private email on her gym's blog two days later, along with Glassman's response. Though Glassman had not been the original addressee, on June 5, he wrote (cc'ing nine other people, including Brian Mulvaney),

> Alyssa,
> I sincerely believe that quarantine has adversely impacted your mental health.
>
> I won't speak for Jeff Cain [whom Alyssa had mentioned in her email as calling her the "conscience of CrossFit" due to her work on queer athlete inclusion] but I can tell you that you are delusional in thinking that anyone even for a second thought that you were "the conscience of CrossFit." The very notion is cringe-worthy.
>
> You think you're more virtuous than we are. It's disgusting. Your self-professed brand wizardry has been tolerated but never seen as actually thoughtful or effective, but certainly manipulative.
>
> You're doing your best to brand us as racist and you know it's bullshit. That makes you a really shitty person. Do you understand that? You've let your politics warp you into something that strikes me as wrong to the point of being evil.
> I am ashamed of you,
> Greg

Alyssa used a screenshot of the email as the header image on her gym's blog post, writing, "I think it really says all that needs to be said about their response when called out. The gaslighting, the belittling . . . The rest of this blog post will be the letter that was sent to Brian, the CEO. It is our blueprint for why we are disaffiliating." Alyssa's blog post made the CrossFit rounds on June 5. Two days later, already enmeshed in fights with affiliate owners, enraged by the nationwide lockdown due to "stay-at-home orders" issued by the US government or via local or state orders, and having been a longtime skeptic of governmental health organizations (as in his attacks on Big Soda, for example), Glassman posted a tweet that would change his life forever.[26]

On June 7, 2020, the Institute for Health Metrics and Evaluation (IHME), like so many others, was voicing its opinion that racism is wrong *and* a public health problem. A now famous tweet read, "Racism and discrimination are critical public health issues that demand urgent response." The tweet also included the trending hashtag #blacklivesmatter, a link to the director of the IHME's official statement on racism as a public health issue, and a large black rectangle with white lettering that read, "Racism is a Public Health Issue." That same day, Glassman, with his blue checkmark and @CrossFitCEO handle, replied, "It's FLOYD-19." He followed up that tweet with a longer one in the early hours of June 8: "Your failed model quarantined us and now you're going to model a solution to racism? George Floyd's brutal murder sparked riots nationally. Quarantine alone is 'accompanied in every age and under all political regimes by an undercurrent of suspicion, distrust, and riots.' Thanks!" A 9 p.m. June 8 tweet on the CrossFit main Twitter page tried to walk back some of Glassman's comments, quoting him: "@CrossFitCEO: 'I, CrossFit HQ, and the CrossFit community will not stand for racism. I made a mistake by the words I chose yesterday. My heart is deeply saddened by the pain it has caused. It was a mistake, not racist but a mistake."

But the damage was compounded on June 9 when BuzzFeed shared a leaked recording of a Zoom call in which, hours before Glassman's "FLOYD-19" tweet, he told affiliate owners, "We're not mourning for George Floyd—I don't think me or any of my staff are." In this leaked audio, he asked a Minneapolis gym owner who had questioned why the brand had not posted a statement about the protests across the country after the death of George Floyd, "Can you tell me why I should mourn for him? Other than that it's the white thing to do—other than that, give me another reason."[27]

Shortly after the publication of the BuzzFeed story, CrossFit announced that Glassman was stepping down as CEO and "retiring." "On Saturday I created a rift in the CrossFit community and unintentionally hurt many of its members," Glassman wrote. "I cannot let my behavior stand in the way of HQ's or affiliates' missions. They are too important to jeopardize."[28]

But the damage was done. Many gyms decided to disaffiliate. The number kept shifting, but it seemed that a few thousand were changing their names. Games athletes, led by Katrin Davidsdóttir, denounced CrossFit HQ, and associated brands distanced themselves. Reebok, one of CrossFit's most famous brand collaborators, cut ties.[29] Reebok issued a statement to *CNN Business* on June 8: "Our partnership with CrossFit

HQ comes to an end later this year. Recently, we have been in discussions regarding a new agreement; however, in light of recent events, we have made the decision to end our partnership with CrossFit HQ. We will fulfill our remaining contractual obligations in 2020." On Facebook, Rogue also distanced itself from CrossFit, writing in a statement quoted by *CNN Business* on June 8 that Rogue "plans to reevaluate its work with the company going forward. 'Rogue does not support the latest statements made by the CrossFit CEO, Greg Glassman. His comments are unacceptable under all conditions.'"[30]

The next two weeks would see more brands distance themselves from CrossFit, affiliates drop CrossFit from their gym names, and elite or famous CrossFitters, including Jason Khalipa (the winner of the Games whom Glassman had stated was "evidence" of the CrossFit method, which had made him the "fittest person on Earth"), and Rich Froning (a devoted Christian and winner of the Games both as an individual and as part of a team), publicly denounce Glassman's statements and claim disaffiliation because it was "Time for Change."[31]

It was hard to keep up with the fallout.

Soon after the maelstrom regarding racist comments came an eruption of revelations about the sexist culture of CrossFit HQ cultivated by Glassman. On June 12, a former CrossFit HQ employee (Glassman's pilot) and decorated Navy SEAL with five Bronze Stars and a Purple Heart named Andy Strumpf used his podcast, *Cleared Hot*, to discuss his time at HQ and all the things he saw and heard.[32] In the YouTube version of the podcast, he sits on his deck with a lake and wilderness background and a pile of chopped wood on his left. He asks of anyone who was also there who wondered if they did the right thing, "Put your mother, or your sister or your wife, or your daughter into the same events or situations you saw play out over time and tell me if you would be comfortable sitting back and being unwilling to speak up." He says that he is not a fan of drama and that he knows that he will see fallout for taking a stand against CrossFit and Glassman. In fact, in the first few minutes of the episode, he attests to how much CrossFit has saved his life but declares that he has to say something. He has to do the right thing.[33]

On June 20, the *New York Times* published an article titled "CrossFit Owner Fostered Sexist Company Culture, Workers Say." Therein, Katherine Rosman writes,

When Greg Glassman resigned earlier this month as chief executive of CrossFit, Inc., excoriated for comments about George Floyd's death on Twitter and in a Zoom meeting, people who have worked there were surprised that his downfall was tied to accusations of racism.

They had assumed that the reason would be routine and rampant sexual harassment.

Interviews with eight former employees, and four CrossFit athletes with strong ties to the company, reveal a management culture rife with overt and vulgar talk about women: their bodies, how much male employees, primarily Mr. Glassman, would like to have sex with them and how lucky the women should feel to have his rabid interest.[34]

Rosman's story goes on and on detailing many terrible #metoo moments.

On June 24, the *New York Times* published another Katherine Rosman story, titled "Greg Glassman, Embattled Owner of CrossFit, to Sell His Company." In it, we learn that the fallout from his racist comments and the years of sexual harassment was causing Glassman to sell his company. Glassman, the cocreator/founder, CEO, and sole owner of CrossFit, who had litigiously held on to CrossFit through various legal battles and a bitter divorce, buying out his ex-wife, Lauren Jenai, in 2012, was forced out.[35] Dave Castro had found the perfect buyer: Eric Roza, a tech billionaire, a CrossFit gym owner, and a CrossFitter since 2008—or, as Castro called him, "one of us."[36]

On June 26, a new Instagram account named "blackatcf," with a black fist as its cover image and identified as a space that is "not affiliated with CrossFit Inc." and in which "all the experiences are gathered anonymously," posted twenty-seven times. The posts were all on a black background with white lettering, some with one slide and others with multiple slides, each testifying to what it feels like to be Black (or a person of color) at CrossFit. These included being subject to racist comments, such as being told by a (presumably white) CrossFit coach that "Black people weren't really made to do CrossFit, unfortunately," and racist undercurrents, such as when someone wrote that they hold their breath when the music starts, hoping the lyrics are edited so they "don't have to engage with folks about why they can't say n**ga" when they are "really just trying to workout," and just a general white supremacist ethos in the gym, much like that in the United States, as one person wrote: "The CrossFit community is supposed to be special. I suppose it is for some. But when you're Black, it hits different. It's simply a microcosm of American society. You're allowed, but never invited. Maybe accepted, but never embraced. And once you get a little too Black, or speak up a little too forcefully, they turn their back on you. 'Y'all can stay here, just as long as you don't make anybody uncomfortable.'" On and on the stories went, giving voice to the range of Black experiences at CrossFit and expressing thanks for a "safe space" to speak their "traumas" and be heard.

Less than three weeks after Glassman's original tweet, he was no longer part of CrossFit. It was a whirlwind of events, and stories and information circulated in many different ways—through news articles in the *New York Times*, *CNN Business*, and the CrossFit news source *Morning Chalk Up*; via individual CrossFitters or gyms posting on Instagram, Twitter, or their gym's webpage; in podcasts revealing long-held secrets; in leaked Zoom recordings; and in text chains, direct message (DM) conversations, and lots of second- or third- or tenth-hand knowledge. It was an anthropologist's dream and nightmare. It was impossible to follow every lead or thread.

But this turmoil in CrossFit was not because of one problematic tweet, a mean email, or Glassman's remarks about George Floyd in Zoom calls. CrossFit and its culture have always been exclusive, violent, and fear based, despite the narrative of inclusion that CrossFit tells about itself. As we have seen, violence and white supremacy are also part of the culture of CrossFit, especially in the United States, infused into the everyday practice of the regimen and highlighted by CrossFit's annual spectacle, the CrossFit Games. CrossFit emerged in the early 2000s, shortly after the 9/11 terrorist attacks and the beginnings of the war on terror. Glassman began training elite US combat forces and emergency personnel for the intense circumstances they found themselves in. This training focused on cultivating extraordinary and unknown feats of strength, control, and stamina through the "methodology" of varied (unknown) and functional movements (real-life movements demanded on the battlefield rather than the gym, e.g., pull-ups versus biceps curls) performed at high intensity (extraordinary feats during life-or-death situations). CrossFit was birthed and raised in the nursery of violence and death in response to fears of terrorism from outside, nonwhite intruders.

The entire CrossFit methodology, which was the saving grace of CrossFit itself when many people were distancing themselves from the brand through disaffiliating their gyms, is a fitness system and culture that glorifies war, death, and hegemonic masculinity, a masculinity that lionizes toughness and competitiveness. The officially named CrossFit workouts are almost exclusively named after fallen US soldiers from the war on terror, or they are female names, "The Girls," deliberately reminiscent of how the weather service used to name high-intensity, potentially destructive storms with female names. All the named workouts except the numbered ones, named for CrossFit Games workouts, are linked to violence, death, and destruction. CrossFit is intended to prepare the body and mind (and heart?) for some unknown violent catastrophe. Though some CrossFitters are indeed former or active military, most are white Americans with postgraduate educations and household incomes over $150,000. Arguably, those who are able to pay a couple of hundred dollars a month for a gym membership are unlikely to be the ones who see their children off to war or to be poor people of color.

In my own visits to many CrossFit gyms, I have seen only a handful of Black people, Indigenous people, or other people of color. Some of these individuals have told me explicitly how they must constantly negotiate their nonwhiteness in the CrossFit space. Even if there are Black people, Indigenous people, and other people of color who participate in CrossFit, it seems clear that, despite all the claims about being an inclusive "community" or the local flavors gyms take, CrossFit gyms remain white spaces that nurture a community based on the values of toughness, competitiveness, and individualism in response to an upended social world such as the COVID-19 pandemic. The community they create is forged from violence and fear and is most likely to feel inclusive if you are elite and/or white.

Most non-CrossFitters know CrossFit because of the ESPN-televised CrossFit Games, which has made CrossFit more of a household name. As we have seen, despite the claim that the Games provide "global representation," almost all the athletes are white. It is overwhelmingly white people competing to be the fittest on Earth, with a handgun as the winner's prize. It is hard not to call to mind eugenics claims about racial fitness and white superiority. Violence and whiteness are celebrated by CrossFit. Many progressive CrossFitters and affiliates wrestled with this reality. Some left with heavy hearts, as CrossFit had changed their life, but they valued inclusiveness. More conservative affiliates forged ahead under the CrossFit banner unsure what all the fuss was about. I did not think that the "shit hitting the fan" that CrossFitters have been preparing for would come from something Glassman would say. It will take a different kind of fitness to survive CrossFit's self-made apocalypse.

Off/on the Couch

In a 2017 YouTube video, Greg Glassman tells a group of people at a CrossFit coaches training courses how CrossFit can transform someone's life and health, moving them from sickness to fitness. CrossFit can lead to better health measures, such as better blood pressure or bone density levels and so on, and to a reduction in the risk of chronic disease. Simply put, one's risk of chronic disease, or what Glassman calls the "independent variable," is "lifestyle choices of what you fuckin ate and what you did for exercise. That's it. That's the problem. It's also where the solution lies. The solution is off the carbs and off the couch."[37] CrossFit has long tried to get people off the carbs and off the couch. CrossFit encouraged people to find a CrossFit gym, scale the workout (modifying it to one's own fitness levels), follow a "paleo" diet, and "count macros." (Recall that Glassman told Alfonsi on *60 Minutes* that he "invented that doing lateral raises and curls while eating pretzels is dumb.") If they do this, they will find their way, through agony and laughter, community and discipline, pain and gains, from "sickness" to "wellness" to "fitness," a continuum that one learns about in CrossFit's Level 1 course, which is required to become a CrossFit coach.[38]

During the pandemic in 2020 and especially while under government stay-at-home orders, many people, especially those in professional or managerial careers, found themselves on the couch, eating the carbs, with their gyms closed. This was the exact opposite of the "unknown unknowns" that CrossFitters had been preparing for as they trained for the apocalypse. CrossFit's preparation was for war, disaster, catastrophe. When "shit hits the fan," CrossFitters are prepared to be heroes, to scale walls, row marathons, fight off zombies, and outfitness whatever came their way. But shit hit the fan in 2020 when COVID-19 coursed through hospitals, towns, countries, and continents and caused millions of deaths, millions of hospitalizations, and massive disruptions to social lives, incomes, and global supply chains due to worldwide lockdowns, even for those who did not become sick. CrossFitters were not prepared for the public health response to the global pandemic: to stay on the couch.[39]

In May 2020, the biological anthropologist Cara Ocobock and I conducted a survey on stay-at-home orders, fitness regimens, and perceptions of well-being, including physical and mental health. We had over five hundred people respond to our survey thanks to social network sampling, including a call for respondents by *Morning Chalk Up*, a CrossFit news source. We found out many things, as the data were robust and insightful. But one of the most interesting things we found was that women were significantly more resilient in their fitness practices than men were.[40] Their resilience was correlated to their exercising in groups before the pandemic. They followed this group-oriented practice during the stay-at-home orders. They met up outside and exercised together. They got online and worked out as a group. While this resilient group was mostly women, it also included some CrossFit men, as they also tend to exercise in a class-based setting. We found that those who had exercised in groups before the stay-at-home orders and gym closures fared much better overall.[41] Yet despite faring better overall, CrossFitters still suffered during the pandemic's stay-at-home orders. Many wanted nothing more than to get back into the gym. They were losing all their gains, they wrote on the survey, and nothing compared to the intensity of the classes.

In some CrossFit circles, the global shutdown stirred resentment. On November 20, 2020, a CrossFit affiliate owner in Buffalo, New York, made national news by facing off with his local sheriff and health department—a vigilante protecting his rights and his land against "the law." A video posted on YouTube showed the gym owner and a crowd of over one hundred people get rowdier and rowdier and end up chasing the officials out.[42] On November 24, the gym owner was interviewed on Fox News, where, on national television, he ripped up fines he had incurred for not following the gym closure restrictions.[43] Dave Castro, the Navy SEAL who is known for his work on the CrossFit Games and who has held many positions at CrossFit HQ, including interim CEO when Glassman "retired," reposted the Fox News video along with the hashtag

#supportyourlocalbox. We would come to learn that earlier in the year, the same gym owner responded to a Buffalo woman who wanted her money back from an event that had been canceled in January but was being held in July in defiance of lockdown orders with an email that read, "I will refund your money as soon as you eat my ass you filthy, foreign, third-world country piece of shit. Fuck you very much." This email would come to light in November via the WNYMedia Network.[44]

In Alyssa Royce's blog post, she cited a "Fluffy Duck" meme, in which a white, youngish (late twenties, early thirties) man sits on his couch in a large living room with a television remote in his hand and a frown on his face, wearing a T-shirt that reads, "Kinda Fit Kinda Fluffy," a slogan of the Fluffy Duck brand, which, according to its website, sells "funny CrossFit and gym shirts."[45] Alongside him is a pillow with the image of the New England Patriots and a whiteboard that reads in magnetic letters, "Some guy eats a bat halfway around the world and now I can't go to CrossFit." The meme had been shared on the official CrossFit social media accounts that Royce had called "problematic" with "racist" messaging.

These are just two examples of the radical CrossFit responses to gym closures and stay-at-home orders that many countries implemented as a public health response to the pandemic. This focus on "public" health and the call for those who could stay at home to do so, to protect those in their communities who were more at risk of death or serious complications from the virus, was at odds with the "off the couch" mantra and the neoliberal understanding of health that CrossFit espouses: you and your lifestyle choices alone are what cause your chronic disease, and those chronic diseases put you at risk of COVID-19 complications—or more simply, you alone are responsible for your health, including dying of COVID-19, and your choices should not impede mine.

It was this neoliberal perspective on health that Glassman had been lecturing on, or shouting about, for years, if not decades. He found the public health response, the stay-at-home-for-others call from the US government an infringement on his libertarian-infused rights. His second post on the Institute for Health Metrics and Evaluation's Twitter page said as much: "your failed model quarantined us." While the lockdown ended up causing serious social strife in the United States due to our rugged individualism and neoliberal tendencies in so many areas of life, not just fitness or CrossFit, it did save lives—millions of lives by some estimates. But the demonizing of the public health response in general and the infectious disease expert Anthony Fauci, who served as one of the lead and most visible members of the White House Coronavirus Task Force, in particular by some people on the right obscures the real lifesaving results of stay-at-home orders.

Stay-at-home orders were not the disaster, catastrophe, or "war" that CrossFitters had been training for. Every single element of CrossFit stood in stark contrast to the public health demands of the pandemic: stay at home for your less fortunate nonwhite neighbors. The violent, contrarian, intense, in-your-face elements of CrossFit did not readily incorporate caretaking for others. The white supremacist, hegemonic masculine, individualistic, Christian, imperialist values of CrossFit were the opposite of those needed during the pandemic. And when faced with this kind of apocalypse, this "unknown unknown," this "shit" that was hitting the fan, CrossFit training did not help at all. In fact, it hurt many of those who devoted themselves to it, from the original CrossFitter Greg Glassman to the Buffalo gym owner to many people of color and women who had found a way to stick with CrossFit despite all their nagging feelings or the overt racist or sexist tendencies of others. In 2020, the monster coming for CrossFitters was not a zombie but a deadly virus that was easily spread and the racism and sexism experienced by many people in their gyms.

Conclusion

While Glassman did not talk about the apocalypse, his overzealous resistance to mainstream health mandates and to the Black Lives Matter movement seemed like his cult-leader downfall during what felt like the end times in American society. Some people followed his call for resistance to mainstream or government-led guidance, often with deleterious effects, such as gym closures.[46] But not everyone did; Glassman could not mobilize his members. While many had blindly followed him through years of misogyny, making excuses or looking the other way, as Strumpf claims he did, CrossFit's libertarian model also allowed for dissenting voices or freedom of thought against Glassman. Devoted CrossFitters echoed many of the elements of Glassman's cult-leader-like hubris and saw their own downfall from their self-sacrificial following. But not all of them. The preemptive email from Alyssa Royce or the rapid backlash against Glassman for his comments reveals the freedom that many CrossFit gyms and their owners have in the affiliate organizational structure.

In a news article for BuzzFeed, Spencer Mestel illustrates how COVID-19 and stay-at-home orders effectively split CrossFit in two.[47] On one side were those who were defying government lockdown orders, including Marjorie Taylor Greene, the onetime CrossFit gym owner and avid CrossFitter turned congresswoman who trained in a gym with others during the pandemic, and the Buffalo New York gym owner. On the other side were thousands of gym owners, dozens of elite Games athletes, and many individual CrossFitters who decided that enough was enough and that they were done with the CrossFit brand after Glassman's racist remarks and the coming to light of his long history of misogyny and sexual harassment.

The fracturing of CrossFit could have been predicted based on the work of Miranda Joseph, who writes "against the romance of community."[48] She comments that often the framework of "community" is used to mobilize one identity and, in so doing, fails to consider other elements of who people are. The "CrossFit community" is supposed to elevate the CrossFit identity among those who identify with it in contrast to other identities, such as Black, liberal, conservative, feminist, LGBTQ+, or Christian. During this tumultuous time in CrossFit's history, the other elements of people's identities came into direct opposition to the CrossFit one, thereby causing fault lines where these tensions had always been. During relatively prosperous and calm times, the tensions were obscured by the call to community. But when "shit hit the fan," the "romance" of the CrossFit community was shattered, breaking it into various factions that had always already been present. This fracturing was painful because the loyalty to CrossFit's beloved community was there. That loyalty could withstand the affiliation with Christian settler-colonial violence in the regimen and ideology. However, it could not take the in-your-face violence of George Floyd's death or the racism of Greg Glassman, who did not really care about such police violence. Once the fault lines along CrossFit's whiteness were exposed, the patriarchal misogynic tensions were also made visible. And the house came crashing down.

Matt Hart writes in his July 2023 *New Yorker* article "Does CrossFit Have a Future?," "All of the CrossFit Games athletes who had denounced Glassman returned to compete this past October. Of the three hundred gyms that had threatened to de-affiliate, less than half followed through. Nicole Carroll [one of CrossFit HQ's longest-tenured employees, who had resigned in early June 2020] even returned to her role as the head of the CrossFit seminar business."[49] With Glassman gone, many people devastated by what happened to CrossFit during 2020 found a way back to the brand, the regimen, the community to which they were devoted. They had not drunk the Kool-Aid with Glassman. Maybe CrossFit could be saved. Maybe Roza, the new owner, would lead them all home.

Conclusion

It is November 2023, and I am meeting my friend at one of the CrossFit gym in Brooklyn that was my home CrossFit gym for two years but I have not been to in months. I watch as the ten o'clock class warms up. There are still a ton of people in the class, all sweating profusely and breathing heavily. The American flag still hangs in the corner. The CrossFit banners from the days of Regionals still hang, as do the official CrossFit posters showing the progression of the press, push press, and push jerk.

My friend and I go across the street to another garage, the same gym but without the structured class and no official coach on duty. She and I are working out side by side. I am training for an Olympic weightlifting competition, and she is preparing for Wodapalooza, an international CrossFit competition held in Miami every year.[1] My friend was aiming to compete for the third time in January 2024. Each time she competed in a team division with friends. We were two of twelve in Open Gym, the garage space filled with people doing their own workouts, training for a special event, performing weird movements, all knowing how to use the defiantly barren gym space. None of us would have felt as comfortable in a mainstream gym. But none of us were doing the official CrossFit class. Nonetheless, we felt right at home.

I have been to this CrossFit gym a handful of times since it reopened after the end of pandemic restrictions. Old friends have left, moved out of the city, or started doing other fitness regimens. Some coaches have left. Some have married. Others are delighted to be back at the gym after a few months traveling the world. One world traveler told me, "I've really missed helping people. It was fun, but I'm happy to be home, excited to do what I love." The gym owner is turning forty, and no one can believe it. Wasn't he still in his early twenties? He has owned and operated this CrossFit gym for fifteen years, and he and it, like the rest of us, seem to have matured.

The gym's vibe is a bit different, calmer. People write less on the blog, perhaps because the most prolific writers no longer go to the gym. The leaderboard is now gone; the gym is less focused on competition and tracking the best times and numbers. This gym has always been inclusive of artists, nonathletes, foodies, and hipsters. It is Brooklyn, after all. But it seems a bit more so now. Perhaps the lack of focus on competition is because of the pandemic and the trauma that many people in New York endured due to all the death and sickness; perhaps they also want to count the pleasure of the workouts now. Maybe the competition seems less fierce because we are all a bit older, slower, smarter. Mortal. The best athletes have left and moved to the suburbs to raise their children or are doing more running and biking than CrossFit classes. They are trying to be a bit more holistically fit rather than simply CrossFit fit.

CrossFit HQ is also calmer. It is not making headlines as much anymore. It has been a few years since CrossFit's implosion and the selling of the company to the tech billionaire Eric Roza. Roza established a diversity, equity, and inclusion division before he moved from CEO to board chairman. There was the firing and quick rehiring of Dave Castro, but even that seemed to be less messy than the Glassman days. The "Battles" tab on CrossFit's main website is gone, probably jettisoned with Glassman, who took his battles with him. The official website still posts WODs, but it has more "normal"-looking people on the webpage; fewer look like the Games superheroes. I have tried to access old webpages using links from older newspaper articles on the beefs that CrossFit and Glassman had. They are all gone, replaced with a "That's a No Rep" webpage, using CrossFit slang to tell me that those pages did not make the transition. There is less red on the website and more blue. I find this quieting; I wonder if this is the intended effect. CrossFit, like the rest of us, seems to have grown up or settled down. We all have less to prove, perhaps, and are just trying to stay sound.

Just Another Exercise Regimen?

When I was in India studying CrossFit in 2018, I noticed that many fitness trends were booming alongside CrossFit. Running events, such as 5ks or half marathons, were only a few years old. Fancy gyms with cardio and weight machines were also new, popping up to fill the fitness needs of the new and giant Indian middle class. Supplement shops and stores selling chicken were also new, catering to the new protein-conscious fitness enthusiasts. What struck me was how new much of the fitness landscape was, not just CrossFit.[2] CrossFit was one of many new ways people were getting healthy or losing weight. It did not have the combative vibe or competitive edge that I had found ubiquitous in the United States.

When I was in Australia that same fall, I became a member of one of Melbourne's first CrossFit gyms. It was known as the home of the second fittest man in Australia and a team that always went to the Games. There were official named banners across the gym illustrating how elite the members were, as those banners were from Regionals or the Games. It was there that the head coach made us all do strict everything during WODs. We were not allowed to kip, an explosive movement from the hips using momentum, anything; we had to do strict pull-ups in workouts. Even burpees, we had to do with strict push-ups rather than flopping ourselves down on the ground. The vibe of the gym was different from what I encountered in the United States. Sure, everyone was competing; Australia is known for its sporting culture and CrossFit prowess. But, as I was point-blank told, "We don't do the weird military stuff. You all [meaning Americans] are a bit fanatical about that stuff." "That stuff" was the Hero WODs undergirded by the ideology of American CrossFit, in which training was linked to disaster and war. Instead, the CrossFit in Melbourne was more for sport. People used it to be better at rugby, Australian rules football, or CrossFit, not in relation to zombies or an apocalypse. The strict stuff would make us better in sports or competition; we were not Navy SEALs training for unknown unknowns.

I had also done CrossFit in France, Morocco, Peru, and Hong Kong, and in each place outside the United States, the "vibe" of CrossFit was less end of days and more "let's get a good workout in" and "do better than last time." There was less at stake, it seemed. Even in the Melbourne gym, where people were super-elite, the vibe was less violent, less angry. The cross in CrossFit was not about salvation or even about being cross as in angry (as someone at a lecture I gave thought the "cross" of CrossFit meant); it was more like the "cross" in "cross-training." This cross-cultural experience put into stark relief how *American* the anger, violence, salvation, and cultiness of CrossFit was in the United States. As

I experienced CrossFit outside the United States, I realized that I needed to return home and find out where that "American stuff" came from. This book on cultural Christianity is my answer.

Today, CrossFit in the US feels a bit more like the CrossFit in other parts of the world was prepandemic: less angry, less redemptive, less culty, more like another fitness practice, more like a place to see your friends and get your sweat on, but less like one's life is at stake or one's soul needs saving.

In fact, in December 2023, a gym owner told me that he saw a CrossFit posting on LinkedIn that used an image of someone sprawled out on the floor, Christ-like on the cross, to promote CrossFit as an everyday fitness regimen. While this is a classic CrossFit pose, this gym owner tells me, "That's not the message we should still be sending!" He used the word "still" to mark that yes, it might have worked once, but it does not anymore. CrossFit should not be about going brutally hard to meet up with Pukey the Clown or Uncle Rhabdo but to fight against chronic disease. He finished that sentence with, "But no one asked me." If you asked him, which I did, he thinks CrossFit should be promoting more general fitness: "Get people in the gym, get them sweating, spike their heart rate a few days a week, but, most importantly, just get them moving." "Don't destroy them," he tells me; that just is not a "mature" message. He owned a mature gym and wished CrossFit HQ would more consistently act mature.

Another gym owner told me that he does not even worry about what HQ is doing: "I don't really know who is up there. No one at my gym would know about Glassman or Castro. I had a [famous CrossFitter] come to my gym, and no one knew who he was. I just run a business to get people to exercise. Politics doesn't come up much. Everyone gets along, even people who are getting divorced right now." When I asked him if any of the new changes that Roza had implemented were useful to him, he said, "The early get-togethers with gym owners in the area was good. They also have a regional rep who would help out. But not really." I asked him if the CrossFit name deterred people from his gym, as it did for Alyssa Royce. He did not think so. "I don't think more than 1 percent of people know about CrossFit," let alone the crazy saga of 2020. He said, "People want a good workout, to be done in an hour, and to see their friends." His gym provides that in a CrossFit class setting. But no one is going to the Games, no one is paying attention to the beefs, and no one knows or cares if Glassman is there or not.

The legacy for these gym owners is really about "health and fitness" and "strength and conditioning." It is to get people off the couch and on the right amount of carbs. Does it help people? Yes, of course it does. Does it save their life? Sure, from the chronic disease coming for most American adults and in much the same way that any regular exercise could help save someone's life. But not in the culty way, not to push yourself so hard that you find yourself in a pain cave looking for the promised land or on the frontier mobilizing righteous (self-)violence to vindicate your claims.

CrossFit claims to be unconventional, mobilizing a new method of fitness and community that sought to change the world. It was created by a self-identified rogue personal trainer who claimed that the fitness revolution was taking place in the garage. But for all the unconventional hype, CrossFit is really conventional. It builds on common American tropes, national narrative projects, like the frontier and the garage as unconventional spaces for innovation. This is a classic American entrepreneurial origin story. The frontier, as the location of the next big thing, is as American as apple pie. It also builds on classic narratives of American superheroes, vigilante white men who save the day, their communities, and themselves through redemptive "righteous" violence. This narrative taps into underlying codes of patriarchal, white supremacist, settler Christian colonial frameworks that shape stories of America and its place in the world. There are also endless stories of salvation through CrossFit, mapping onto normative templates of the narrative arc of redemption for many Americans. How much more conventional can you get? What CrossFit did was *market* itself as revolutionary, as anti-"the man" or big business because Americans like nothing more than a rogue revolutionary (vigilante) who will stick it to the man (the "Law"). But it did so using national narratives and underlying codes left in the wake of white Protestant Christianity. CrossFit uses convention to locate the good life and the classic American quest for it in Christianity's wake, in its many afterlives.

Also, CrossFit is fantasy. The idea that it is rogue or revolutionary is not reality. The idea that CrossFit is based on science—physics or evolutionary—is a fantasy. It is marketed as physics but does not actually measure any physical quantities. It is marketed as based on primordial human functional capacities and tapping into genetic potential, but there is little scientific basis for these presumptions and proclamations. It is fantasy to believe that there is "one human diet" that will reveal one's "genetic potential." But isn't that what marketing is: selling fantasy to those who believe it as real? CrossFit also mobilizes other American fantasies such as the national narrative projects of hard work and meritocracy, that everyone is on the same equal playing field. However, due to settler Christian colonialism, this is not and has not ever been true. As Christina Sharpe argues, Black people in the diaspora, including the United States, live in the wake of slavery.[3] Its legacies are not passed; they erupt in the present, as Saidiya Hartman lists the ways: "skewed life chances, limited access to health and education, premature death, incarceration, and impoverishment."[4] Sharpe also calls for *thinking* in the wake (wake work) to disrupt these violent pasts that have not passed, to imagine an otherwise from what we know about the continued afterlives of slavery.[5] Therefore, I *think* all of us live in the wake of slavery and settler Christian colonialism that continues to sharply divide those for whom the American Dream's fantasies work and those for whom they do not. In addition to the good life, by examining how cultural Christianity operates in our supposedly secular society, we can see how other ideologies such as militarism, white supremacy, patriarchy, and capitalism are violent afterlives of a violent white Protestant Christianity that took root in the New World and still leaves its wake. Could we imagine an "otherwise"?[6]

CrossFit's Legacy

In 2021, Matt Hart interviewed Eric Roza about his ownership of CrossFit and his desire to bring it back from the brink following CrossFit's 2020 reckoning, including CrossFit's confrontation with its racist and misogynist roots, Glassman's departure, and the COVID-19 pandemic. Roza wants CrossFit not only to survive but to thrive by having one hundred million people doing CrossFit by 2031. This depends on the success of the local gyms, the quiet heroic coaches, the Games athletes, and the people looking to get and stay fit. Roza tells Hart, "I didn't do this for the money. The reason I'm doing this is because I'm completely in love with CrossFit and I want to bring it to other people."[7] Roza echoes Oprah in using his love as a driving motivator for capitalist gain, but he does not have the guru identity. Roza also does not have the dogmatic ferocity of Glassman. Nor does he have Glassman's libertarian values.

Right after I finished interviewing the CrossFit gym owners about their relationship with CrossFit HQ and the post-2020 fitness landscape, CrossFit HQ informed the affiliate owners that it would raise the annual fee to use the CrossFit name from whatever they were paying to a universal US$4,500. Those who were grandfathered in at $1,000 had to pay $4,500; those in India, Peru, or Morocco (or anywhere) had to pay US$4,500. This policy change set off another firestorm. CrossFit gym owners balked at the increase because Glassman had refused to increase the annual fee once it reached $3,000. Recall how he was against "rent extraction." Furthermore, as social media posts lamented, gym owners said that CrossFit HQ did not do anything for the local affiliates. A new Instagram account was created: CFAC, or CrossFit Affiliate Collective. It was created by affiliate owners who want to take "collective action" to "protect the community" they love. This was not, they posted, a "hostile takeover of HQ," a "coup d'etat," or simply a "financial decision." Rather, it was about "principles," about "getting rid of the pirates" (i.e., venture capitalists) who want to "rent-extract" from local gym owners and not give them anything in return. In a video pinned to the first spot on the CFAC home page, Greg Glassman, the prodigal son returned, states, "Here is what I would do, I would cheerlead for a group who would want to buy [CrossFit] back for affiliates." Perhaps this is a form of what Livia Stone calls "autogestión": collective self-management that is currently finding purchase among people everywhere to resist the exploitation experienced by so many in present-day capitalism.[8] Autogestión is the CrossFit gym moving from the Lyceum to the new gym as everyone takes a load or a group class clearing out the gym to host a wedding. It has the flavor of the spirit of the frontier, where collective effort was required to build cabins and school buildings. But can it go beyond helping just members of the CrossFit gym?

Early on in my research, I told a colleague about the end-times rhetoric used in the CrossFit gym. She asked, "Are they training to be able to take their wheelchair-bound or elderly neighbors out of a burning building?" I did not know the answer at the time but inquired further as the research developed. After seven years of investigation, I have an answer: No, not really. CrossFit training is about self-preservation, or if it is collective, it is about a team of super-fit people surviving together. Cross-

Fitters are not really looking out for the more vulnerable among us. The COVID-19 pandemic revealed this very starkly. In contrast, the anthropologist Lauren Griffith provides a moving examination of capoeira as a physical practice that mobilizes practitioners toward social justice goals rather than only individualistic ones.[9]

It is both fantasy and deeply held beliefs about rugged individualism based on white exceptionalism that lead someone to believe that they can survive the end times (or even rent increases) through their own physical capacities or independent will. The reality is that we need each other; CrossFit affiliates need each other. White people are not exceptionally built to withstand an apocalypse or even neoliberal capitalism alone. We need collectives to stand up to venture capitalists. We need to stay home to not spread a deadly virus. The end times will require that we take care of each other. The only way to actually deal with such catastrophic events is to mobilize together rather than react as lone vigilante superheroes. If we are to live in the wake of Christianity, perhaps we can live in the wake of those elements of the religion that demand inclusion of the poorest and most vulnerable, that argue that rich "pirates" will see not heavenly reward, or that violence is not the answer no matter how righteous ones claims that it is.

It remains to be seen what will happen with CrossFit. Will affiliates remain loyal to the brand? Will they leave? Will CrossFit continue in its current trajectory and become more like other fitness brands and US companies, beholden to the shareholders, who wield supreme power in US capitalism? Or will local gym owners unite and mobilize against it, akin to other such organizing efforts that the United States has seen in the past several years (such as the unionizing efforts of Starbucks and Amazon workers) but predicated on historical workers' rights and small-business-owner movements? CrossFit, like other aspects of American society, seems to be awakening to the violence of the afterlives of its slavery and settler Christian colonialism through its racisms, militarism, capitalism, patriarchy, and misogyny.[10] Instead of assuming that the US is a secular nation, perhaps it is time to come clean about the wake of the cultural Christianity that Americans live in. If we do, perhaps we can live otherwise with care and nonviolence (actual life, liberty, and the pursuit of happiness?), collective action (actual democracy?), and social justice (actual equity and humanity?) for all.

ACKNOWLEDGMENTS

I am grateful to everyone I had the pleasure of working with on this project. A big thank-you to all the CrossFitters out there who told me their story, let me work out next to them, and included me in the party. I am awed by your commitment to each other, especially during the pandemic that ravaged our world. Thank you to the gym owners who always found time to answer my questions and the gym coaches for always pushing me along the way. I learned a lot from everyone I met—from Brooklyn to Albuquerque to Delhi to Melbourne—and my life has been changed forever.

My work was undergirded by my colleagues at Brooklyn College. First, to my colleagues in the Department of Anthropology—Patricia Antoniello, Kelly Britt, Jillian Cavanaugh, Stephen Chester, Shahrina Chowdhury, Meghan Ference, Leticia Medina, Kelsey Pugh, Rhea Rahman, and Naomi Schiller: thank you for your support, goodwill, and collegiality. We have such a great group. Big thanks to Elise Goldberg in the Children and Youth Studies Program especially during the end times of this project; our ship never sank. Thank you to Dr. Lauren Mancia, a historian and scholar of Medieval Christianity, who included me in a variety of events so that I could ask different kinds of scholars about the Christianity I saw happening in CrossFit. I especially appreciated our Faculty Day panel "Religion in Unexpected Places," where Dr. Mancia, Dr. Andrew Arlig (philosopher of metaphysics), Dr. Timothy Shortell (sociologist of religion), and other members of the Brooklyn College faculty shaped my thinking on cultural Christianity. Thank you to Professor Arthur Bankoff (chair of Anthropology), Dean Kleanthis Psarris (dean of the School of Natural and Behavioral Sciences), and Provost William Tramontano for the funding for gym memberships during this research project. I could not have done this without it. Thank you to Dean Peter Tolias, the current dean of the School of Natural and Behavioral Sciences, for his support of this project too. The publication of this book was made possible by two generous grants from the Tow Foundation at Brooklyn College.

Also, thank you to the PSC-CUNY for funding to complete this book. The generous support of Brooklyn College—in so many ways—made the completion of this book possible. I am very grateful.

I am also grateful to the Wenner-Gren Foundation for funding the Anthropology of Anxiety project. My intellectual engagement with Nutsa Batiashvili, Stéphanie Larchanché, Susan Lepselter, Rebecca Lester, Townsend Middleton, and Saiba Varma on anxiety transformed this book in profound ways. Thank you all for your insights and encouragement. During a visit to Georgia for the Anthropology of Anxiety, Nikoloz Aleksidze began what would become a long conversation about Christianity, including schisms from antiquity to the present day. I am grateful to him for the hours of knowledge sharing and for always answering my questions with deep historical and cultural context.

Thank you to Washington University in Saint Louis's Department of Anthropology, which hosted an Anthropology of Anxiety conference in April 2023. I shared early drafts of chapters in the Ethnographic Theory Workshop, and the insights from those events shaped my thinking. I want to give an extra thank-you to James Wertsch for the gift of his book and his detailed read of my chapters. Your scholarship has profoundly shaped the way I think about stories, narrative, and underlying codes. Thank you for shaping my intellectual growth.

Also thank you to the University of California, San Diego, for inviting me to share my initial thoughts on CrossFit at its Psychological and Medical Anthropology Seminar Series. Those early questions from Professors Thomas Csordas and Janis Jenkins set this book on the right path; thank you. Thank you to Cara Ocobock and the University of Notre Dame for funding the Strong A(s) F(eminist) conference. It brought together scholars from the collaborate project *Gender and Power in Strength Sports* (2023), and I learned a great deal about CrossFit from people studying it in other parts of the world, including Alessia Mastrorillo, Riikka Turtiainen, and Usva Friman. Thank you to Noelle Brigden and Melissa Forbis for their collaboration in that project; you shaped my insights here.

I want to thank the experts who reviewed the specialized knowledge in this book. This includes Dr. Timothy McGee, Dr. Nikoloz Aleksidze, Dr. Earl Y. Thorpe Jr., Dr. Cara Ocobock, and Dr. Craig A. Robin. I learned more nuance and detail about various kinds of Christianity, pain caves, Dante, physics, Neanderthal diets, and primate locomotion from your expertise than I could have imagined. Thank you for your time and efforts on this project.

Thank you to Livia Stone, Nutsa Batiashvili, and Stéphanie Larchanché for Writing Group (and beyond). The regular sharing of our writing has been a source of much pleasure in my life. Your nuanced questions and insights at various stages of the book's development were crucial for its completion (and my sanity). I could not have done this without you, especially there at the end. I deeply value our friendship and collegiality. Thank you, Liv, for your insightful comments during your much-needed breaks. Thank you to Earl Y. Thorpe Jr. for his detailed reads and intellectual engagement in this project. Your help was vital, especially at the end stages; I am very grateful for you. Thank you to Sharon Lennon for her television script writer's eye and mind; this book's story is indebted to your reads. Thank you to Jeanne Hejtmanek for your assistance in the footnotes and bibliography; your efforts made for a smoother finish.

Thank you to Jennifer Hammer at New York University Press for her support and dedication to this project. Thank you for your detailed revisions and consistent encouragement. Also, a huge thank-you to the external reviewers of this book: your thorough and thoughtful feedback was crucial for honing my argument.

Thank you to Coach (Juan) Blanco and my teammates, including Matthew Andrade, Veta Bates, Andrew Chen, Kelly DeLear, Alba Fortuna, Lucie Gehringer, Monica Knowlton, Siera Schuster, Tony Schuster, and Ajeet Seenivasan, at Brooklyn Training Hall. I love lifting heavy, and I love doing it with you all. A special thank-you to Monica Knowlton for her efforts on my bibliography and her daily loving push in the gym.

Finally, thank you to my family for their support of my work. I was able to live with Jenny Hejtmanek, Craig, Milada, Mira, Macy, Hub, and Wesley during the pandemic, and my life was made whole therewith. Thank you, Milada and Mira, for letting me into your lives. I love you more than words can describe. Thank you to my parents, Jeanne and Mike Hejtmanek, for their constant support, encouragement, and love. I appreciate all you do and have done. Thank you to my brother, Michael Hejtmanek, and his family, Kim, Harper, and Sadie, for their constant long-distant support. I feel it. Thank you.

Despite all this intellectual and moral support, any and all errors in this book are mine.

GLOSSARY

AMRAP: A workout with a specific time clock, such as fifteen minutes, and one does as many rounds as possible (AMRAP).

BURPEE: A dynamic exercise in which one moves from standing to a plank to a push-up to a squat, finishing with a jump.

BOX: The colloquial name given to a CrossFit gym, as it resembles a box and is in contrast to the "big-box" gyms such as Bally's or Lifetime Fitness.

CROSSFIT: A trademarked brand cofounded by Greg Glassman and Lauren Jenai.

DOUBLE-UNDERS: A jump-rope skill in which the rope goes under the feet twice with each jump.

HERO WODS: Workouts named after US soldiers and service members who have died, usually during combat and in the war on terror.

FOR TIME: A workout that is done as fast as possible.

FRAN: One of "The Girls." It consists of the workout scheme of 21-15-9 thrusters and pull-ups.

GIRLS, THE: Workouts named like the National Weather Service used to name storms with female names.

KIP: The use of hip power and momentum to do upper-body movements, such as pull-ups. The result is kipping pull-ups, which allow for more pull-ups to be done faster in a workout.

METCON: Metabolic conditioning, the timed part of the workout.

MURPH: A Hero WOD named after the Navy SEAL Lieutenant Michael P. Murphy. It is usually performed on Memorial Day in CrossFit gyms in the United States.

THRUSTER: A barbell skill in which the barbell is caught in a deep squat and then is thrust overhead.

TOES-TO-BAR, OR T2B: a skill where one holds onto and hangs from a pull-up bar and brings one's toes to the bar and then back down, often they are done with a swinging or kipping motion.

21-15-9: A rep scheme that usually includes two exercises in which each exercise is done twenty-one times, then fifteen times, and finally nine times. It originated with Fran.

WOD: Workout of the day.

NOTES

CrossFit is a registered trademark of CrossFit, Inc. The opinions and analyses expressed in this book are solely the author's and do not reflect the opinions of CrossFit, Inc.

INTRODUCTION

1. CBS News 2015.
2. Mastrorillo 2023.
3. Dawson 2017.
4. Maguire 2008.
5. This is in line with scholarly definitions as well, including those found in Durkheim 1995; Geertz 1973; Lofton 2017; Weber 1930.
6. See, for example, Hefferman 2008b; Musselman 2022; Burton 2018; Thurston and ter Kuile 2015.
7. Weber 1930.
8. Sharpe 2016.
9. Wertsch 2019.
10. Sharpe 2016, 3.
11. Sharpe 2016, 9.
12. Others use "the wake" to understand various aspects of racialized live in the United States; for an example in education and pedagogy, see Adkins Hernández and Muñoz de Luna 2021.
13. Brand 2001, 25.
14. Hartman 2008, 6.
15. This is not the same as being secular. Cody Musselman (2022) argues that CrossFit is a postsecular activity because it brings in elements of the religious, and this makes sense for some elements of CrossFit. However, I think a better way to think about CrossFit and the way Christianity works in the United States is through Sharpe's work on the wake, Brand's understanding of history, Hartman's concept of afterlives, and Wertsch's framework of underlying codes. I think the framework of postsecular relies too much on formal religion being part of nation-state legal practices (Asad [1982] 1993, 2003; Casanova 1994, 2006; Crockett 2018; Habermas 2008), and I am more focused on popular culture and the ubiquity of cultural Christianity outside of legal parameters.
16. I am not arguing about the separation of church and state, a hallmark of modern societies and therefore secular states. Much like Talal Asad (2002), I think that despite overt claims of secularism, the United States, built on the foundation of Christian values and cosmology, could never really be secular; its laws were inherently produced by Christians. Asad even argues that one of anthropology's most

popular definitions of religion is inherently a Christian framework, as it is based on the heritage of the author Clifford Geertz, an American.
17 Wertsch 2019.
18 Throughout this book, I use pseudonyms and composites of people to protect anonymity as much as possible. Some of the data are in the public realm, so names are used then. It is standard practice to alter names and/or to use composites when writing up anthropological data. This project was approved by the CUNY Institutional Review Board (IRB) #2016-0580.
19 I had not ever used this framing. I used "being in shape" or "being fast," but this phrase never sounded normal when I said it. I think CrossFit made "being fit" and "fitness" more popular in general.
20 Bourdieu 1977; Foucault 1988; Mauss 1973.
21 Csordas 2002.
22 Csordas 2002, 244.
23 Farnell 2012.
24 For other anthropology on sport using this method, see Bar-On Cohen 2009; Csordas 1990; Downey 2007; Pavlidis and Fullagar 2015; Spencer 2009.
25 Marc Boglioli had been studying hunting in Vermont before this project; see his book Boglioli 2009.
26 Boglioli, Hejtmanek, and Stroupe 2002.
27 Intimately informed by Dunbar-Ortiz 2018.
28 Infogram, n.d.; Rally Fitness 2017.
29 See, for example, Osorio 2014; or Reynolds 2022.
30 See Heywood 2015; Knapp 2015a; and Washington and Economides 2016.
31 See, for example, Murphy 2012.
32 Beyond the Whiteboard 2015.
33 Chidester 2005.
34 Besnier, Brownell, and Carter 2018, 1.
35 Petrzela 2016.
36 Honkasalo 2001; J. Jackson 1994; Lelwica 2017.
37 See, for example, Bedchel 2021; Caillois 2001; Cederström and Spicer 2015; Dworkin and Wachs 2009; Spielvogel 2003.
38 Weber 1930; Tocqueville 1838.
39 Tocqueville 1838, 303.
40 C. Smith 2003, 1.
41 Pew Research Center 2014.
42 For a discussion of the relationship between religion, secularism, and modernity as organizing frameworks for nation-state construction, see Asad 2003. There are also considerable debates about Western nations being postsecular; for an examination of these debates, see Habermas 2008; Crockett 2018; and Casanova 1994, 2006.
43 Kivel 2013, 3. See also Fessenden 2007; and Moore 2003.
44 See, for example, Preston 2012; Rodgers 2018.

45 MacIntyre 2007, 219.
46 As I do this, I build on the work of Marcelle Dawson (2017) and her understanding of CrossFit as a reinventive institution.

CHAPTER 1. A CULT, A COMMUNITY, A RELIGION RUN BY A BIKER GANG

1 Musselman 2022.
2 Feuerherd 2016.
3 Higgens 2012; Klippenstein 2013.
4 I write about a "zombie apocalypse" framing in Hejtmanek 2020.
5 Cooperman 2005.
6 Clifford 2016.
7 Hefferman 2008a, 2008b.
8 Thurston and ter Kuile 2015.
9 Harvard Divinity School 2015.
10 Fields 2013.
11 Schulson 2017.
12 One Church 2013.
13 Lange 2021.
14 Ulrich 2016.
15 Chidester 2005, viii.
16 Chidester 2005, viii.
17 Chidester 2005, 3.
18 Musselman 2019, 626.
19 Musselman 2022, 176.
20 Musselman 2022.
21 R. Griffith 2004; Putney 2001.
22 Petrzela 2022, 16. See also Green 1986.
23 Green 1986.
24 Lelwica 2017.
25 Green 1986; R. Griffith 2004; Lelwica 2017; Petrzela 2022.
26 R. Griffith 2004.
27 R. Griffith 2004, 249.
28 R. Griffith 2004, 250.
29 Black 2013, xiii.
30 Macfadden and Oswald 1903, 11.
31 Luther 2011. See also Black 2013.
32 See also Waller 2011.
33 R. Griffith 2004, 70.
34 Putney 2001. See also Ladd and Mathisen 1999.
35 Putney 2001, 2.
36 Ultimate Performance 2021; Merrill 2022.
37 Putney 2001. See also Ladd and Mathisen 1999.

38 Lelwica 2017.
39 Froning with Thomas 2013. See also Hodges 2013.
40 Bunch 2012.
41 FAITH RXD, n.d. (emphasis in original).
42 No one who filled out a questionnaire for me identified any religious affiliation.
43 Instagram post, December 11, 2021.
44 Instagram post, March 8, 2019.
45 I am guilty of this. I have argued that the zombie apocalypse was a secular version of the apocalypse; see Hejtmanek 2020. It comes off as secular, but it is based on Christian and biblical themes.
46 Musselman 2024, 235.
47 McCloud 2004.
48 Barker 2014, 236.
49 Barkun 1993, 597.
50 Musselman 2024.
51 Atkin 2004, xiv (emphasis in original).
52 Musselman 2024. See also Raynsford 2021, 94.
53 Musselman 2024, 245.
54 Musselman 2024, 243.
55 Musselman 2024, 241–246. See also CrossFit Inc. 2009a; Walsh 2006; r/CrossFit 2019.
56 CrossFit Inc. 2005.
57 CrossFit Inc. 2022.
58 Herz 2014; Heywood 2016.
59 Oldenburg 1989.
60 Sarason 1974.
61 Pickett et al. 2016.
62 Simpson et al. 2017.
63 V. Turner 1967, 1969.
64 E. Turner 2011, ix.
65 Thurston and ter Kuile 2015, 10.
66 Glassman 2017a.
67 Glassman 2017b.
68 His mother, Sarah Royce, wrote an autobiography at the request of her son Josiah. It tells the story of an American pioneer woman during California's Gold Rush: S. Royce 1932.
69 J. Royce 1886; Gilpin 2017.
70 Gilpin 2017, 3.
71 J. Royce 1899.
72 J. Royce (1913) 1968, xxv (emphasis in original).
73 J. Royce (1913) 1968, 67.
74 J. Royce (1913) 1968, 68.
75 J. Royce (1913) 1968, 95.

76 Herstein 2009, 101.
77 Joseph 2002, viii.
78 Hells Angels MC World, n.d.
79 Barger, Zimmerman, and Zimmerman 2000, 2002. See also Wolf 1991.
80 Barger 2000.
81 See, for example, Knapp 2015b; and Kerry 2016.
82 Beynon 2023.
83 M. Hay 2018; Bowles 2015.
84 Cooperman 2005.
85 Wise 2000.
86 Ta 2006.
87 Palahniuk 1996, 51.
88 Hejtmanek, under review.

CHAPTER 2. SALVATION THROUGH BEARING ONE'S DAILY CROSS(FIT)

1 I consulted with two historians of religion about the use of testimonials, including the scholar of medieval Christianity Lauren Mancia and the scholar of antiquity and Eastern Christianity Nikoloz Aleksidze.
2 Augustine (401) 2008.
3 Gilden 2019; Tuveson 1968.
4 Gilden 2019.
5 Gilpin 2017.
6 Glucklich 2001. For an examination of the "secularization" of pain, see Caton 1985.
7 Glucklich 2001, 13, 40, 29, 200, 21.
8 I have been informed by Earl Y. Thorpe, an African American pastor, that this pain and suffering in American Christianity is associated with white American readings of Christian history and white American Christian theology. Black American Christian life takes on liberation theology frameworks more so than pain and suffering.
9 Perkins 1995, 13.
10 These new narratives and the suffering self are in conversation with two contemporaneous frameworks of the body and self. One is the Stoics, a Greco-Roman philosophical tradition that instructed its followers to "master and ignore" the body's claims. The suffering self was set in contrast to this philosophical tradition. The second, and complementary, framework was that of Galen and his medical understanding of the body, which prioritized monitoring and deciphering an interior life to better understand oneself. Both frameworks—Stoicism and Galen's—thrived during the same early centuries of the Common Era (CE) (Perkins 1995).
11 This focus on pain also includes arguments against the experience of pain. Stephanie Cobb (2016) suggests that martyrs may not have experienced pain; rather, they emulated Christ's impassibility, and modern readers project pain onto contemporary readings of hagiographies.

12 Markschies 2007, 352.
13 Perkins 1995, 39–40.
14 Perkins 1995, 142.
15 Glucklich 2001, 23.
16 Glucklich 2001, 25.
17 The study of pain crosses disciplinary boundaries, from scholars studying athletes' pain experience and tolerance (Pettersen, Aslaksen, and Pettersen 2020) to psychoanalysts investigating people who are drawn to pain (Freud 1962) to medical anthropologists examining narratives of pain associated with illness (J. Jackson 1994) to religious scholars exploring meanings in voluntary pain (Daniel 1984; Glucklich 2001) to cultural theorists (Scarry 1985).
18 International Association for the Study of Pain, n.d.-b.
19 International Association for the Study of Pain, n.d.-a.
20 Good et al. 1992; J. Jackson 1994; Honkasalo 2001.
21 Cobb 2016, 16.
22 Nuñez 2020.
23 See also Kassel, n.d.
24 For additional descriptions of pain caves, see Hejtmanek, under review.
25 The book of Jonah is a teaching parable, a fable, understood as such by those who would hear it. Like many teachings of the Hebrew Bible, Christians have attached many interpretations and meanings to the famous "whale" and Jonah, forgoing the satirical nature of the story and missing the meaning of God's mercy toward humanity, even the brutal Assyrian empire. What remains clear is the adaptation of the story as miraculous to many people in Christian teaching. From that understanding, a point of departure extends to various interpretations (many demonstrably wrong) that extend from this story. What remains is an ardent belief in the actors and plot of the story by Christians with a less tangible hold on the actual meaning and comprehension of the narrative. Thus, you see Marcia using the imagery of the whale not because of the theological import but because of the imagery that many of the Old Testament stories provide. Christians tend to map onto the imagery of the story more than the theological underpinnings. This instructive interpretation provided by Earl Y. Thorpe.
26 I want to thank Tim McGee and Nikoloz Aleksidze for their assistance in interpreting Marcia's pain cave description.
27 Hell having three gates is also referenced in the Hindu text the Bhagavad Gita. However, Marcia identifies as a former Christian who was raised in an American Protestant church, complete with visits to church camp. Therefore, her references here are formally Christian and culturally Christian rather than Hindu.
28 Borawski 2015.
29 McAdams 2008, 20.
30 McAdams 2006.
31 Gilpin 2017, 2, 1.
32 Gilpin 2017, 1, 5.

33 These Protestant notions are also informed by Catholic theology and imagery, as it is challenging to separate all of the elements into neat, distinct story lines. For an examination of how American literature mixes and separates Protestant and Catholic stories, see Fessenden 2007.
34 See, for example, Margaret Mead's *Coming of Age in Samoa* (1928), which was an investigation of adolescence outside the United States to provide evidence that adolescence was not experienced the same everywhere, that the American theories of "storm and stress" were not a universal, biological human condition (see Hejtmanek, forthcoming).
35 To be fair, Talal Asad (2002, 125) argues that Clifford Geertz's widely accepted definition of "religious belief" is a "modern, private Christian one."
36 For more on the psychological revolution that secularized American public life, see Meador 2003. See also James 1890, 1902.
37 Lelwica 2017; R. Griffith 2004.
38 Perkins 1995, 142, 39–40.
39 Glucklich 2001, 29.
40 Cooperman 2005.
41 Calder, n.d.
42 M. Hay 2018; Cooperman 2005.
43 For a discussion of Fran Lung, see Hejtmanek, under review.
44 Cooperman 2005.
45 Ulrich 2016.

CHAPTER 3. CROSSFIT CAPITALISM

1 Glassman 2013.
2 Glassman 2013 (emphasis added).
3 Glassman 2013, comment 1.
4 Glassman 2013, comment 2.
5 Glassman 2013, comment 4.
6 Glassman 2013, comment 10.
7 Glassman 2013, comment 13.
8 Glassman 2013, comment 30.
9 Henderson 2018.
10 Glassman 2012 (emphasis added).
11 Peck 2010, 8. See also Lofton 2006; Peck 2008.
12 Peck 2010, 8.
13 Peck 2010, 8.
14 Lofton 2011, 5.
15 Starker (1989) 2008, 8.
16 Starker (1989) 2008, 14–15.
17 Starker (1989) 2008, 18.
18 Elkins 2017.
19 See also Ashoff 2015.

20 Lofton 2011, 25.
21 Lofton 2011, 45, 235.
22 Hutchinson 2014.
23 For more information on church polity, see Gaustad and Schmidt 2002; Youngs 1998.
24 Ornella 2015. See also Ornella 2019.
25 For more information on pilgrim badges, see de Kroon 2004.
26 Lemay 2013.
27 Petrzela 2022, 311.
28 Erlanger and Govela 2018, book jacket, 5 (emphasis in original).
29 Erlanger and Govela 2018, 43.
30 Erlanger and Govela 2018, 97, 138.
31 Erlanger and Govela 2018, 142, 168.
32 Glassman 2002a.
33 Glassman 2002a, 1.
34 Glassman 2002a, 10.
35 Dreshare, n.d.
36 Erlanger and Govela 2018, 14.
37 Glassman 2005, 1.
38 Glassman 2005, 2.
39 Erlanger and Govela 2018, 146.
40 Glassman 2005, 4–5.
41 Erlanger and Govela 2018, 170.
42 Erlanger and Govela 2018, 90.
43 Rogue Fitness, n.d.
44 Rogue Fitness, n.d.
45 Foster 2019.
46 Vennare, n.d.
47 McKenzie 2013.
48 Cooper 1968.
49 Masco 2014.
50 Glassman 2007.
51 Musselman 2019, 626.
52 Hejtmanek 2023.

CHAPTER 4. CROSSFIT AND THE AMERICAN FRONTIER SPIRIT

1 Slatta 2001, xiii. This serves in contrast to Roxanne Dunbar-Ortiz's (2018) *Indigenous Peoples' History of the United States*, in which violence was not righteous but ruthless and totalizing.
2 For a more complete history of the United States from an Indigenous perspective, see Dunbar-Ortiz 2018. See also Grenier 2005.
3 Library of Congress, n.d.
4 O'Sullivan 1839.

5   This white male suffrage was forged through the genocide of many Indigenous people and entire civilizations; see Dunbar-Ortiz 2018, chap. 6.
6   Turner's thesis contrasted with evolutionary notions of the day, what was called "germ theory," or that habits and characteristics are inherent and racially determined. Turner argued that environment shaped these attributes of people and peoples, not "germs" passed down through ancestry. See Billington 1958.
7   For more on this process, see Wagner 2025.
8   Of course, I am focusing on the myth of the frontier, rather than the actual, detailed history. This myth is whitewashed to limit the known ruthless violence that these settlers enacted against Indigenous peoples throughout the contemporary United States; for a more complete history rather than mythology, see Dunbar-Ortiz 2018.
9   Billington 1958, 86–89.
10 Nor could they form militia groups to destroy Indigenous villages and kill Indigenous people without banding together; see Dunbar-Ortiz 2018.
11 Billington 1977, 77. See also Billington 1966.
12 Billington 1977, 84.
13 Slotkin 1973, 1985, 1998.
14 Militias and settler-rangers were prevalent throughout colonization and nation-building in the contemporary United States. In fact, the idea of "irregular warfare," in which militia or rangers are sent in to do what a regular army could not, has deep roots in the US; see Dunbar-Ortiz 2018; and Grenier 2005. Here I focus on popular myths.
15 National Guard, n.d.
16 Slatta 2001, 311.
17 Slotkin 1998, 4.
18 ReasonTV 2013.
19 Petrzela 2022.
20 Brooklyn CrossFit, n.d.
21 W. Jackson 1977, 14.
22 Lundskow 2022, 967.
23 Lundskow 2022, 967. See also Dunbar-Ortiz 2018, 7.
24 Lundskow 2022, 980.
25 Slotkin 1998.
26 Masco 2014.
27 CrossFit Inc. 2009b.
28 Kupper 2023.
29 Kupper 2023
30 CrossFit Inc., n.d.
31 CrossFit Inc., n.d.
32 CrossFit Inc., n.d.
33 Achauer 2014, 3.
34 Hejtmanek 2023.

35 Hejtmanek 2023, 133.
36 Achauer 2015.
37 Lemmon 2017.
38 Pipes 2016.
39 Pipes 2016.
40 Achauer 2013a.
41 Learned Handle 2017.
42 Over twenty thousand people signed a petition to have the prize removed, but Castro replied, "Unless the state and federal laws regarding gun ownership in California and the U.S. change in the next week, then no, nothing is changing." You can find the petition in Bartels 2016.
43 ABC News 2016.
44 Wagner 2025, 30–31.
45 Dunbar-Ortiz 2018, 15.

CHAPTER 5. HEROES AND SHEROES

1 Jung 1981.
2 Campbell 1949.
3 Lawrence and Jewett 2002, 6.
4 Lawrence and Jewett 2002, 6.
5 Mills 2014, 1.
6 Jewett and Lawrence 2003, xiv.
7 Mills 2014, 1 (emphasis in original).
8 Guynes and Lund 2020, 3.
9 Meenan 2022.
10 Hejtmanek 2023.
11 Guynes and Lund 2020.
12 Powers and Greenwell 2017, 535.
13 Demers 2022.
14 Demers 2022.
15 For an exploration of Superman and Nietzsche's Übermensch, see Ojimba and Yammeluan 2019; Schwartz 2022.
16 McNulty, n.d.
17 Rogers 2023.
18 Hughes 2016.
19 World Population Review 2023; Blennerhassett 2020.
20 Washington, and Economides 2016, 153.
21 Guynes and Lund 2020. See also Benson and Singsen 2022.
22 Guynes and Lund 2020; Aman 2022.
23 Izadi 2019. See also Morrison 1992; Guynes and Lund 2020.
24 Jennings 2011.
25 Musselman 2020.

26 Ladd-Taylor, n.d.
27 Wiese 2023.
28 Achauer 2013b.
29 Achauer 2013b, 9.
30 Achauer 2013b, comment 9.
31 Achauer 2013b, comment 6.
32 Lundskow 2022, 980.
33 Washington and Economides 2016, 143.
34 Heywood 2015, 30.
35 Knapp 2015a, 2015b.
36 Turtiainen and Friman 2023, 40.
37 Turtiainen and Friman 2023, 40.
38 Turtiainen and Friman 2023, 47.
39 Trujillo 1991.
40 Kerry 2016.
41 Balaban 2021; *CrossFit Journal* 2004.
42 Johansson 1996.
43 Sen 2023.
44 Ocobock 2023.
45 angels_egg 2016.
46 Glassman 2010c, comment 5.
47 Glassman 2010c, comment 18.
48 Glassman 2010c, comment 26.

CHAPTER 6. SCIENCE, CROSSFIT STYLE

1 Glassman 2002a. In fact, my brother-in-law has his own garage gym and purchased the mats at the local horse-feed store.
2 This contrasts with AMRAP workouts, which are "as many rounds as possible" for a specific amount of time, say, twenty minutes. The person finishing first completed the most rounds when time was up.
3 Rapisarda 2020. I have modified the overview for clarity and length; italics added for emphasis.
4 Beyond the Whiteboard, n.d.
5 Merry 2011, S90.
6 Power 1996, 292.
7 Shore and Wright 2015, 424.
8 Shore and Wright 2015.
9 Strathern 1996–1997, 13.
10 Glassman 2002b.
11 Glassman 2010a.
12 I consulted Craig A. Robin, who has a PhD in optical science and engineering and has served as the senior research scientist for directed energy applications at the

US Army's Space and Missile Defense Command and director of the Directed Energy Project Office at the US Army's Rapid Capabilities and Critical Technologies Office. He is now the CEO of EO Solutions, a physics and engineering company.
13 Glassman 2010b.
14 Glassman 2010a, comment 44.
15 Glassman 2010a. If you look into the team of world-class scientists at CrossFit, you quickly learn that the chief science officer is Jeff Glassman, who does have a PhD in science systems and has been identified as a "rocket scientist." But he is also Greg's father, the same man who made Greg measure a thousand nails to the nearest thousandth of an inch, instilling a lifelong lesson about bell curves (or Gaussian distribution) and "that careful observation, coupled with measurement, can reveal secrets of the universe hitherto unknown, unseen, and undiscovered" (Herz 2014, 22).
16 Glassman 2002b.
17 Glassman 2002b.
18 Hejtmanek 2020.
19 Glassman 2002b.
20 Glassman 2010a, comment 65.
21 Glassman 2010a, comment 49.
22 CrossFit Inc. 2012.
23 R. Wolf, n.d.
24 Amenabar and O'Connor 2022.
25 Rossillo 2022.
26 Pobiner 2018.
27 Ocobock, Lacy, and Niclou 2021, 270.
28 Barr et al. 2022.
29 Dalton 1904, 82.
30 Musselman 2020.
31 Glassman 2010b.
32 Berger 2018.
33 Berger 2018.
34 Retraction Watch 2017.
35 Chedekel 2016.
36 Carpenter 2018.
37 Easter 2018.
38 Elshakry 2010.
39 Latour 1988.
40 Pronger 2002. See also Hejtmanek and Ocobock 2022.
41 Gusterson 1998, 225.

CHAPTER 7. THIS WAS NOT THE APOCALYPSE WE TRAINED FOR!
1 Crockett and Zarracina 2016; Boluk and Lenz 2011.
2 Hejtmanek 2020.
3 Hay 2020b.

4   Holte 2020b, xi–xvii; Hay 2020a; Wessinger 2009.
5   Hay 2020b, 6.
6   I will be painting with broad strokes, as the general story is important, but specific details should be sought elsewhere, including Holte 2020a; Sutton 2014; and Wessinger 2009.
7   Sutton 2014, 14.
8   There is of course debate over these details among premillennialist and between pre- and postmillennialists, among white evangelicals and between white and Black American Protestants. In other words, I write as if there is one story of Armageddon when in fact there is not. But for the sake of understanding all the unfolding of apocalyptic ideology, there must be some sort of story from which to begin.
9   Sutton 2014, 18.
10 Sutton 2014, 27.
11 Sutton 2014, x.
12 Sutton 2014, 360.
13 Green 1986. Harvey references the Second Coming and fitness practices in "Part I: Millennial Dreams and Physical Realities, 1830–1860."
14 Sutton 2014, 372.
15 Sutton 2014, 372, 351, xiv.
16 The end-times frameworks are also understood through denominational lines within mainline Protestantism (e.g., Methodist, Lutherans, and Episcopalians) that cut across racial lines. Catholics understand the end-times framework, which also cuts across racial lines within Catholicism (e.g., Latin and African Catholic populations).
17 Sutton 2014, 63.
18 These racialized evangelical Christian frameworks of the end times map onto what happened during the pandemic when the calls for staying at home to help save nonwhite neighbors were resisted or ignored by many evangelical white Americans.
19 Hickman 2020.
20 Spry 2020. See also Jones 2003; Roanhorse 2018; M. Smith (1970) 1981.
21 Sutton 2014.
22 It was published in December 2020, but it was written in 2018–2019; Hejtmanek 2020.
23 Donahue 2020.
24 The "CEO" distinction is somewhat murky here. Alyssa emailed Brian Mulvaney as CEO, but Glassman replied and was considered the CEO when the fallout occurred.
25 Royse 2020.
26 Carpenter 2018.
27 Brooks and Mack 2020.
28 CrossFit Inc. 2020.
29 Duffy 2020.
30 Duffy 2020.
31 Tao 2023. The original Froning statement is from June 7, 2020, on Instagram.

32 Marquez 2020.
33 Strumpf 2020.
34 Rosman 2020a.
35 See Helm 2013.
36 Rosman 2020b.
37 CrossFit Inc. 2017.
38 CrossFit Inc. 2021.
39 DeMartini and Willett 2022; Redwood-Brown 2022.
40 Ocobock and Hejtmanek 2023.
41 Ocobock and Hejtmanek 2022.
42 TimWaltonTV 2020.
43 Mestel 2020.
44 WNYMedia Network 2020.
45 Fluffy Duck Shop, n.d.
46 Lofranco 2020.
47 Mestel 2020.
48 Joseph 2002, viii.
49 Hart 2021; Genetin-Pilawa 2020.

CONCLUSION

1 I went to Miami in 2017 to observe what was a gigantic fitness festival over the Martin Luther King Jr. Day long weekend. Thousands of super-fit people in CrossFit T-shirts and body-revealing clothing watched or competed in the event. There were various divisions in true CrossFit fashion, trying to be sure anyone could compete. It went from Elite (in which Games athletes would compete making prescribed, Rx'ed, weights look light), Rx (for those just under the Elites), Scaled (those who had to modify the workouts or who could not do the Rx), Masters (older than forty), Kids and Teens, and Adaptive (which included people who were in wheelchairs, who had prosthetics, or who needed special assistance). This was the first time I had seen the best, the good, the okay, the old, the young, and those who might have been put into the Para or Special Olympics all competing together, in any sport. I have gone to many sporting events in my lifetime, but this was the first where everyone was all together.
2 Although there is a long history of physical culture and sport in India; see, for example, Alter 1992, 2000; Appadurai 1995; Michelutti 2010; Strauss 2005.
3 Sharpe 2016.
4 Hartman 2008, 6.
5 Sharpe 2016, 18. Also, for a theoretical conceptualization of an "otherwise," see King, Navarro, and Smith 2020.
6 For an example of an otherwise, see Carter 2020.
7 Hart 2021.
8 Stone, under review.
9 Griffith 2023.
10 See, for example, Harris 2017.

BIBLIOGRAPHY

ABC News. 2016. "ESPY Awards: Lebron, Dwayne, Carmelo, Chris Speech on Race and Violence." YouTube, July 14. www.youtube.com/watch?v=5GE5oe8wgag.
Achauer, Hilary. 2013a. "Face the Fear: Lessons from Newtown." *CrossFit Journal*, January 25, 2013. http://library.crossfit.com.
———. 2013b. "The War Within." *CrossFit Journal*, February 10, 2013. http://library.crossfit.com.
———. 2014. "Memorial Day Hurt." *CrossFit Journal*, May 23, 2014. http://library.crossfit.com.
———. 2015. "A Soldier's Tale." *CrossFit Journal*, November 4, 2015. http://library.crossfit.com.
Adkins Hernández, Sean D., and Lucía I. Mock Muñoz de Luna. 2021. "In the Wake of Anti-Blackness and Being: A Provocation for Do-Gooders Inscribed in Whiteness." *Curriculum Inquiry* 51 (1): 161–180.
Alter, Joseph S. 1992. *The Wrestler's Body: Identity and Ideology in North India*. Berkeley: University of California Press.
———. 2000. *Gandhi's Body: Sex, Diet, and the Politics of Nationalism*. Philadelphia: University of Pennsylvania Press.
Aman, Robert. 2022. "Whiteness and the Colonial Origins of America's First Superhero: Lee Falk's *The Phanom*." *Journal of Popular Culture* 55:98–117.
Amenabar, Teddy, and Anahad O'Connor. 2022. "TikTok 'Liver King' Touts Raw Organ Meat Diet. He Also Took Steroids." *Stuff*, December 7, 2022. www.stuff.co.nz.
angels_egg. 2016. "Help Me Rename the CrossFit 'Girls' after Heroic Women." r/Feminism, Reddit. www.reddit.com.
Appadurai, Arjun. 1995. "Playing with Modernity: The Decolonization of Indian Cricket." In *Consuming Modernity: Public Culture in a South Asian World*, edited by C. A. Breckenridge, 23–48. Oxford, UK: Berg.
Asad, Talal. (1982) 1993. *Genealogies of Religion: Discipline and Reasons of Power in Christianity and Islam*. Baltimore: Johns Hopkins University Press.
———. 2002. "The Construction of Religion as an Anthropological Category." In *A Reader in the Anthropology of Religion*, edited by Michael Lambek, 114–132. Malden, MA: Blackwell.
———. 2003. *Formations of the Secular: Christianity, Islam, Modernity*. Stanford, CA: Stanford University Press.
Ashoff, Nicole. 2015. *The New Prophets of Capital*. London: Verso Books.

Atkin, Douglas. 2004. *The Culting of Brands: When Customers Become True Believers.* New York: Portfolio.
Augustine. (401) 2008. *The Confessions.* Translated with introduction and notes by Henry Chadwick. Oxford: Oxford University Press.
Balaban, Dusan. 2021. "CrossFit Benchmark Workouts—'The Girls.'" *BoxRox*, August 26, 2021. www.boxrox.com.
Barger, Ralph "Sonny." 2000. "Interview: Born to Raise Hell." *BBC News*, August 14, 2000. http://news.bbc.co.uk.
Barger, Ralph "Sonny," Keith Zimmerman, and Kent Zimmerman. 2000. *Hell's Angels: The Life and Times of Sonny Barger and the Hell's Angels Motorcycle Club.* New York: William Morrow.
———. 2002. *Ridin' High, Livin' Free: Hell-Raising Motorcycle Stories.* New York: William Morrow.
Barker, Eileen. 2014. "The Not-So-New Religious Movements: Changes in 'the Cult Scene' over the Past Forty Years." *Temenos* 50 (2): 235–256.
Barkun, Michael. 1993. "Reflections after Waco: Millennialists and the State." *Christian Century* 110 (18): 596–600.
Bar-On Cohen, Einat. 2009. "Kibadachi in Karate: Pain and Crossing Boundaries within the 'Lived Body' and within Sociality." *Journal of the Royal Anthropological Institute* 15 (3): 610–629.
Barr, W. Andrew, Briana Pobiner, John Rowan, Andrew Du, and J. Tyler Faith. 2022. "No Sustained Increased in Zooarchaeological Evidence for Carnivory after the Appearance of Homo Erectus." *Proceedings of the National Academy of Science* 119 (5): e2115540119.
Bartels, Daniel. 2016. "Asking CrossFit to Cancel Glock Prizes for the Winners of the 2016 CrossFit Games." *Change.org*, July 13, 2016. www.change.org.
Bedchel, Alison. 2021. *The Secret to Superhuman Strength.* Boston: Houghton Mifflin Harcourt.
Benson, Josef, and Doug Singsen. 2022. *Bandits, Misfits, and Superheroes: Whiteness and Its Borderlands in American Comics and Graphic Novels.* Jackson: University Press of Mississippi.
Berger, Russell. 2018. "NSCA 'CrossFit Study' Fraud?" *CrossFit Journal*, March 6, 2018. https://journal.crossfit.com.
Besnier, Niko, Susan Brownell, and Thomas F. Carter. 2018. *The Anthropology of Sport: Bodies, Borders, Biopolitics.* Berkeley: University of California Press.
Beynon, Steve. 2023. "'Looking for a Husband, Boyfriend, Attention': Study Reveals Sexism Faced by Women in Army Special Operations." *Military.com*, August 21, 2023. www.military.com.
Beyond the Whiteboard. 2015. "Memorial Day Murph." *BTWB* (blog), May 24, 2015. https://btwb.blog.
———. n.d. Home page. Accessed July 5, 2024. https://btwb.com.
Billington, Ray Allen. 1958. "How the Frontier Shaped the American Character." *American Heritage* 9 (3): 86–89.

———. 1966. *America's Frontier Heritage*. New York: Holt, Rinehart and Winston.

———. 1977. *America's Frontier Culture: Three Essays*. College Station: Texas A&M University Press.

Black, Jonathan. 2013. *Making the American Body: The Remarkable Saga of the Men and Women Whose Feats, Feuds, and Passions Shaped Fitness History*. Lincoln: University of Nebraska Press.

Blennerhassett, Patrick. 2020. "CrossFit: Do Shorter Athletes Have an Advantage in the Sport?" *South China Morning Post*, July 29, 2020. www.scmp.com.

Boglioli, Marc. 2009. *A Matter of Life and Death: Hunting in Contemporary Vermont*. Amherst: University of Massachusetts Press.

Boglioli, Marc, Katie Hejtmanek, and Nancy Stroupe. 2002. "Ethnohistorical Overview of the Medicine Bow National Forest." White paper. United States Forest Service.

Boluk, Stephanie, and Wylie Lenz. 2011. "Introduction: Generation Z, the Age of Apocalypse." In *Generation Zombie: Essays on the Living Dead in Modern Culture*, edited by Stephanie Boluk and Wylie Lenz, 1–17. Jefferson, NC: McFarland.

Borawski, Becca. 2015. "CrossFit Kids: Divorce and Custody." *Breaking Muscle*, June 18, 2015. https://breakingmuscle.com.

Bourdieu, Pierre. 1977. *Outline of a Theory of Practice*. Cambridge: Cambridge University Press.

Bowles, Nellie. 2015. "Exclusive: On the Warpath with CrossFit's Greg Glassman." *MAXIM*, September 8, 2015. www.maxim.com.

Brand, Dionne. 2001. *A Map to the Door of No Return: Notes to Belonging*. Toronto: Doubleday Canada.

Brooks, Ryan, and David Mack. 2020. "The Head of CrossFit Has Stepped Down after Telling Staff on a Zoom Call, 'We're Not Mourning for George Floyd.'" *BuzzFeed News*, June 9, 2020. www.buzzfeednews.com.

Bunch, Josh. 2012. "CrossFit Faith: The Spiritual Side." *CrossFit Games*, March 14, 2012. https://games.crossfit.com.

Burton, Tara Isabella. 2018. "'CrossFit Is My Church': How Fitness Classes Provide the Meaning Religion Once Did." *Vox*, September 10, 2018. www.vox.com.

Caillois, Roger. 2001. *Man, Play and Games*. Translated from the French by Meyer Barash. Urbana: University of Illinois Press.

Calder, Tony. n.d. "CrossFit Dangers: Top 10 | Uncle Rhabdo and CrossFit." *Best CrossFit Shoes*. Accessed July 5, 2024. www.bestcrossfitshoe.net.

Campbell, Joseph. 1949. *The Hero with a Thousand Faces*. New York: Pantheon Books.

Carpenter, Murray. 2018. "Mr. CrossFit vs. Big Soda: A Profane Fitness Guru's Wonky War with The Soda Industry." *Washington Post Magazine*, June 4, 2018.

Carter, J. Kameron. 2020. "Other Worlds, Nowhere (or The Sacred Otherwise)." In *Otherwise Worlds: Against Settler Colonialism and Anti-Blackness*, edited by Tiffany Lethabo King, Jenell Navarro, and Andrea Smith, 158–210. Durham, NC: Duke University Press.

Casanova, José. 1994. *Public Relations in the Modern World*. Chicago: University of Chicago Press.

———. 2006. "Rethinking Secularization: A Global Comparative Perspective." *Hedgehog Review* 8 (1): 1–2.
Caton, Donald. 1985. "The Secularization of Pain." *Anesthesiology* 62:493–501.
CBS News. 2015. "King of CrossFit." *60 Minutes*, May 10, 2015. www.cbsnews.com.
Cederström, Carl, and André Spicer. 2015. *The Wellness Syndrome*. Malden, MA: Polity.
Chedekel, Lisa. 2016. "Probing Soda Company Sponsorship of Health." *The Brink: Pioneering Research from Boston University*, October 14, 2016. www.bu.edu.
Chidester, David. 2005. *Authentic Fakes: Religion and American Popular Culture*. Berkeley: University of California Press.
Clifford, Catherine. 2016. "How Turning CrossFit into a Religion Made Its Atheist Founder Greg Glassman Rich." *CNBC*. August 28, 2016. www.cnbc.com.
Cobb, Stephanie. 2016. *Divine Deliverance: Pain and Painlessness in Early Christian Martyr Text*. Berkeley: University of California Press.
Cooper, Kenneth, H. 1968. *Aerobics*. New York: Bantam Books.
Cooperman, Stephanie. 2005. "Getting Fit, Even If It Kills You." *New York Times*, December 22, 2005. www.nytimes.com.
Crockett, Clayton. 2018. "What Is Postsecularism?" *American Book Review* 39 (5): 6–14.
Crockett, Zachary, and Javier Zarracina. 2016. "How the Zombie Represents America's Deepest Fears." *Vox*, October 31, 2016. www.vox.com.
CrossFit Inc. 2005. "Workout of the Day: Sunday 051113." November 13, 2005. www.crossfit.com.
———. 2009a. *Every Second Counts: The Story of the 2008 CrossFit Games*. CrossFit Pictures.
———. 2009b. "National War College Speech, Part 1." YouTube, January 6, 2009. www.youtube.com/watch?v=E6yR3kikADc.
———. 2012. "CrossFit Whiteboard: Functional Movement." YouTube, September 14, 2012. www.youtube.com/watch?v=aAaKk1ADccs.
———. 2017. "Greg Glassman: Off the Carbs, Off the Couch." YouTube, October 12, 2017. www.youtube.com/watch?v=Mm5-1IxDTno.
———. 2020. "Greg Glassman Retires." June 9, 2020. www.crossfit.com.
———. 2021. "What Is Fitness? Part 4: The Sickness-Wellness-Fitness Continuum." October 2, 2021. www.crossfit.com.
———. 2022. "What Is CrossFit in Six Words?" http://community.crossfit.com.
———. n.d. "Hero and Tribute Workouts." Accessed July 5, 2024. www.crossfit.com.
CrossFit Full Bore South. n.d. "What Is CrossFit in Six Words??" Accessed July 5, 2024. www.crossfitfullboresouth.com.
CrossFit Journal. 2004. "The New Girls." November 2004. http://library.crossfit.com.
Csordas, Thomas. 1990. "Embodiment as a Paradigm for Anthropology." *Ethos* 18 (1): 5–47.
———. 2002. *Body/Meaning/Healing*. New York: Palgrave Macmillan.

Dalton, Francis. 1904. "Eugenics: Its Definition, Scope, and Aims." *Journal of American Sociology* 10 (1): 82.
Daniel, E. Valentine. 1984. *Fluid Signs: Being a Person the Tamil Way*. Berkeley: University of California Press.
Dawson, Marcelle C. 2017. "CrossFit: Fitness Cult or Reinventive Institution?" *International Review for the Sociology of Sport* 52 (3): 361–379.
de Kroon, M. 2004. "Medieval Pilgrim Badges and Their Iconographic Aspects." In *Art and Architecture of Late Medieval Pilgrimage in Northern Europe and the British Isles*, vol. 1, edited by Sarah Blick and Rita Tekippe, 385–404. Leiden: Brill.
DeMartini, Anne L., and Jennifer B. Willett. 2022. "'We Should Not Have the Same Restrictions as Everybody Else': Southeastern US CrossFit Coaches' Perceptions of COVID-19 Restrictions." *Physical Culture and Sport Studies Research* 97:77–93.
Demers, Paris. 2022. "How Henry Cavill Got RIPPED for Man of Steel! (CrossFit?!)." YouTube, January 27, 2022. www.youtube.com/watch?v=RDIHeCzoTco.
Donahue, Ben. 2020. "How the NFL Responded to the Colin Kaepernick Protests in 2016–2017 and How the League Responded to Athlete Protests during the Black Lives Matter Movement of 2020: A Sport Study, Social Phenomenological Approach." *Sport Journal* 24.
Downey, Greg. 2007. "Producing Pain: Techniques and Technologies in No-Holds-Barred Fighting." *Social Studies of Science* 37 (2): 201–226.
Dreshare. n.d. "Greg Glassman Wiki (CrossFit CEO) Age, Wife, Biography, Family & More." Accessed September 2, 2023. www.dreshare.com.
Duffy, Clare. 2020. "Reebok Cuts Ties with CrossFit after CEO's Controversial Tweets about George Floyd." *CNN Business*, June 9, 2020. www.cnn.com.
Dunbar-Ortiz, Roxanne. 2018. *An Indigenous Peoples' History of the United States*. Boston: Beacon.
Durkheim, Émile. 1995. *Elementary Forms of Religious Life*. Translated by Karen E. Fields. New York: Free Press.
Dworkin, Shari L., and Faye Linda Wachs. 2009. *Body Panic: Gender, Health, and the Selling of Fitness*. New York: New York University Press.
Easter, Michael. 2018. "CrossFit's Greg Glassman Disrupted Fitness. Next, He's Taking on Healthcare." *Men's Health*, October 12, 2018. www.menshealth.com.
Elkins, Kathleen. 2017. "Daymond John and 2 Other 'Sharks' Say This 80-Year-Old Book on Wealth Changed Their Lives." *CNBC Make It*, October 17, 2017. Accessed July 5, 2024. www.cnbc.com.
Elshakry, Marwa. 2010. "When Science Became Western: Historiographical Reflections." *Isis* 101 (1): 98–109.
Erlanger, Olivia, and Luis Ortega Govela. 2018. *Garage*. Cambridge, MA: MIT Press.
FAITH RXD. n.d. "Chapters." Accessed July 5, 2024. https://faithrxd.org.
Farnell, Brenda. 2012. *Dynamic Embodiment for Social Theory: I Move Therefore I Am*. New York: Taylor and Francis.
Fessenden, Tracy. 2007. *Culture and Redemption: Religion, the Secular, and American Literature*. Princeton, NJ: Princeton University Press.

Feuerherd, Peter. 2016. "Drinking the Kool-Aid at Jonestown." *JSTOR Daily*, November 11, 2016. https://daily.jstor.org.
Fields, Leslie Leyland. 2013. "The Fitness-Driven Church." *Christianity Today*, June 21, 2013. www.christianitytoday.com.
Fluffy Duck Shop. n.d. Home page. Accessed June 7, 2020. https://fluffyduckshop.com.
Foster, Tom. 2019. "The Man of Steel behind CrossFit's Favorite Gym Equipment." *Men's Health*, November 8, 2019. www.menshealth.com.
Foucault, Michel. 1988. "Technologies of the Self." In *Technologies of the Self: A Seminar with Michel Foucault*, edited by Luther H. Martin, Huck Gutman, and Patrick H. Hutton, 16–49. Amherst: University of Massachusetts Press.
Freud, Sigmund. 1962. *Civilization and Its Discontents*. Translated by James Strachey. New York: Norton.
Froning, Rich, with David Thomas. 2013. *First: What It Takes to Win*. Carol Stream, IL: Tyndale House.
Gaustad, Edwin, and Leigh Schmidt. 2002. *The Religious History of America*. Rev. ed. New York: Harper One.
Geertz, Clifford. 1973. *The Interpretation of Cultures*. New York: Basic Books.
Genetin-Pilawa, Joe. 2020. "Nicole Carroll Returns; Says 'I Want to Be Part of This Future.'" *Morning Chalk Up*, June 29, 2020. https://morningchalkup.com.
Gilden, Linda. 2019. "What Does Testimony Mean in Christianity?" *Christianity.com*, July 15. www.christianity.com/wiki/christian-life/what-does-testimony-mean-in-christianity.html.
Gilpin, W. Clark. 2017. "American Narratives of Sin and Salvation." *Oxford Research Encyclopedia, Religion*. Oxford: Oxford University Press. https://oxfordre.com.
Glassman, Greg. 2002a. "The Garage Gym." *CrossFit Journal*, September 1, 2002. http://journal.crossfit.com.
———. 2002b. "What Is Fitness?" *CrossFit Journal*, October 1, 2002. https://journal.crossfit.com.
———. 2005. "Garage Gym II: The Revolution." *CrossFit Journal*, July 1, 2005. http://journal.crossfit.com.
———. 2007. "Understanding CrossFit." *CrossFit Journal*, April 1, 2007. http://journal.crossfit.com.
———. 2010a. "Defining CrossFit." *CrossFit Journal*, December 27, 2010. http://journal.crossfit.com.
———. 2010b. "Real Science." *CrossFit Journal*, June 24, 2010. http://journal.crossfit.com.
———. 2010c. "You Are CrossFit." *CrossFit Journal*, January 22, 2010. http://journal.crossfit.com.
———. 2012. "The Founder's Views Part 3: The Business of CrossFit." *CrossFit Journal*, August 3, 2012. http://journal.crossfit.com.
———. 2013. "Pursuing Excellence and Creating Value." *CrossFit Journal*, January 22, 2013. http://journal.crossfit.com.
———. 2017a. "Coach Glassman at Harvard: Creating Culture." *CrossFit Journal*, January 11, 2017. https://journal.crossfit.com.

———. 2017b. "Coach Glassman at Harvard: Laughter and Agony." *CrossFit Journal*, January 11, 2017. https://journal.crossfit.com.
Glucklich, Ariel. 2001. *Sacred Pain: Hurting the Body for the Sake of the Soul*. Oxford: Oxford University Press.
Good, Mary-Jo DelVecchio, Paul E. Brodwin, Byron J. Good, and Arthur Kleinman, eds. 1992. *Pain as Human Experience: An Anthropological Perspective*. Berkeley: University of California Press.
Green, Harvey. 1986. *Fit for America: Health, Fitness, Sport, and American Society*. Baltimore: Johns Hopkins University Press.
Gregory, Sean. 2014. "Lift, Squat, Repeat: Inside the CrossFit Cult." *Time*, January 9, 2014. https://time.com.
Grenier, John. 2005. *The First Way of War: American War Making on the Frontier, 1607–1814*. Cambridge: Cambridge University Press.
Griffith, Lauren Miller. 2023. *Graceful Resistance: How Capoeiristas Use Their Art for Activism and Community Engagement*. Urbana: University of Illinois Press.
Griffith, R. Marie. 2004. *Born Again Bodies: Flesh and Spirit in American Christianity*. Berkeley: University of California Press.
Gusterson, Hugh. 1998. *Nuclear Rites: A Weapons Laboratory at the End of the Cold War*. Berkeley: University of California Press.
Guynes, Sean, and Martin Lund. 2020. "Not to Interpret, but to Abolish: Whiteness Studies and American Superhero Comics." In *Unstable Masks: Whiteness and American Superhero Comics*, edited by Sean Guynes and Martin Lund, 1–16. Columbus: Ohio State University Press.
Habermas, Jürgen. 2008. "Notes on a Post-Secular Society." *New Perspectives Quarterly* 25 (4): 17–29.
Harris, Hamil R. 2017. "U.S. Political Climate Results from 'Theological Malpractice,' D.C. Pastor Says." *Washington Post*, August 25, 2017. www.washingtonpost.com.
Hart, Matt. 2021. "Does CrossFit Have a Future?" *New Yorker*, July 20, 2021. www.newyorker.com.
Hartman, Saidiya. 2008. *Lose Your Mother: A Journey along the Atlantic Slave Route*. New York: Farrar, Straus and Giroux.
Harvard Divinity School. 2015. "CrossFit as Church?!" YouTube, November 16, 2015. www.youtube.com/watch?v=90c8ZRKDCyU.
Hay, John, ed. 2020a. *Apocalypse in American Literature and Culture*. Cambridge: Cambridge University Press.
———. 2020b. "The United States of Apocalypse." In *Apocalypse in American Literature and Culture*, edited by John Hay, 1–14. Cambridge: Cambridge University Press.
Hay, Mark. 2018. "Some CrossFit Gyms Feature Pictures of These Puking, Bleeding Clowns." *Vice*, June 21, 2018. www.vice.com.
Hefferman, Virginia. 2008a. "God's Workout." *The Medium* (blog), *New York Times*, March 23, 2008. www.nytimes.com.
———. 2008b. "Our Warm Up Is Your Workout." *The Medium* (blog), *New York Times*, March 14, 2008. https://archive.nytimes.com.

Hejtmanek, Katie Rose. 2020. "Fitness Fanatics: Exercise as Answer to the Zombie Apocalypse in Contemporary America." *American Anthropologist* 122 (4): 864–875.

———. 2023. "On Death and Fitness: Hero Workouts, US Militarism, and the Necrosociality of CrossFit." In *Gender and Power in Strength Sports: Strong as Feminist*, Critical Studies in Sport Series, edited by Noelle K. Brigden, Katie Rose Hejtmanek, and Melissa M. Forbis, 122–142. Abingdon, UK: Routledge.

———. Forthcoming. "Adolescence and Young Adulthood." In *The Cambridge Handbook of Psychological Anthropology*, edited by Edward Lowe, chapter 12. Cambridge: Cambridge University Press.

———. Under review. "Conjuring and Calming Anxiety: CrossFit and Whiteness in Contemporary America." *American Anthropologist*.

Hejtmanek, Katie Rose, and Cara Ocobock. 2022. "'I Feel Terrible and Need to Exercise to Find Any Sort of Joy': What COVID Stay-at-Home Orders Tell Us about Exercise as Vitality Politics and Entertainment in the United States." *Ethos* 50 (4): 1–14.

Hells Angels MC World. n.d. "The Founding of the Hells Angels Motorcycle Club." Accessed July 5, 2024. https://hells-angels.com.

Helm, Burt. 2013. "Do Not Cross CrossFit." *Inc* 35 (6): 102–116.

Henderson, Scott. 2018. "CrossFit's Explosive Affiliate Growth by the Numbers." *Morning Chalk Up*, October 23, 2018. https://morningchalkup.com.

Herstein, Gary. 2009. "The Roycean Roots of the Beloved Community." *The Pluralist* 4 (2): 91–107.

Herz, J. C. 2014. *Learning to Breathe Fire: The Rise of CrossFit and the Primal Future of Fitness*. New York: Three Rivers.

Heywood, Leslie. 2015. "The CrossFit Sensorium: Visuality, Affect and Immersive Sport." *Paragraph* 38 (1): 20–36.

———. 2016. "'We're In This Together': Neoliberalism and the Disruption of the Coach/Athlete Hierarchy in CrossFit." *Sport Coaching Review* 5:116–129.

Hickman, Jared. 2020. "The Apocalypse of Settler Colonialism and the Case for the Americocene." In *Apocalypse in American Literature and Culture*, edited by John Hay, 17–29. Cambridge: Cambridge University Press.

Higgens, Chris. 2012. "Stop Saying 'Drink the Kool-Aid.'" *The Atlantic*, November 8, 2012. www.theatlantic.com.

Hodges, Wade. 2013. *Train for Something Greater: An Athlete's Guide to Spiritual Fitness*. North Haven, CT: Self-published.

Holte, James Craig, ed. 2020a. *Imagining the End: The Apocalypse in American Popular Culture*. Santa Barbara, CA: ABC-CLIO.

———. 2020b. Introduction to *Imagining the End: The Apocalypse in American Popular Culture*, edited by James Craig Holte, xii–xxi. Santa Barbara, CA: ABC-CLIO.

Honkasalo, Marja-Liisa. 2001. "Vicissitudes of Pain and Suffering: Chronic Pain and Liminality." *Medical Anthropology* 19 (4): 319–353.

Hughes, Robin L. 2016. "All Height Matters: Implicit Bias and Unearned Privileges." *Diverse: Issues in Higher Education*, October 10, 2016. www.diverseeducation.com.

Hutchinson, Dawn. 2014. "New Thought's Prosperity Theology and Its Influence on American Ideas of Success." *Nova Religio: The Journal of Alternative and Emergent Religions* 18 (2): 28–44.
Infogram. n.d. "The Demographics of CrossFit." Accessed July 5, 2024. https://infogram.com.
International Association for the Study of Pain. n.d.-a. "About." Accessed August 2, 2023. www.iasp-pain.org.
———. n.d.-b. "Terminology: Pain." Accessed July 2, 2023. www.iasp-pain.org.
Izadi, Elahe. 2019. "Honoring Toni Morrison through the Words She Shared with the World." *Washington Post*, August 6, 2019. www.washingtonpost.com.
Jackson, Jean. 1994. "Chronic Pain and the Tension between the Body as Subject and Object." In *Embodiment and Experience: The Existential Ground of Culture and Self*, edited by Thomas J. Csordas, 201–228. Cambridge: Cambridge University Press.
Jackson, W. Turrentine. 1977. Foreword to *America's Frontier Culture: Three Essays*, by Ray Allen Billington, 11–17. College Station: Texas A&M University Press.
James, William. 1890. *The Principles of Psychology*. Vol. 1. New York: Henry Holt.
———. 1902. *The Varieties of Religious Experience*. New York: Longmans, Green.
Jennings, Willie James. 2011. *The Christian Imagination: Theology and Origins of Race*. New Haven, CT: Yale University Press.
Jewett, Robert, and John Shelton Lawrence. 2003. *Captain America and the Crusade against Evil: The Dilemma of Zealous Nationalism*. Grand Rapids, MI: William B. Eerdmans.
Johansson, Thomas. 1996. "Gendered Spaces: The Gym Culture and the Construction of Gender." *YOUNG* 4 (3): 32–47.
Jones, Stephen Graham. 2003. *The Bird Is Gone: A Monograph Manifesto*. Tallahassee, FL: FC2.
Joseph, Miranda. 2002. *Against the Romance of Community*. Minneapolis: University of Minnesota Press.
Jung, Carl G. 1981. *The Archetypes and the Collective Unconscious (Collected Works of C. G. Jung, vol. 9, part 1, and vol. 10)*, Translated by R. F. C. Hull, 2nd ed. Princeton, NJ: Princeton University Press.
Kassel, Gabrielle. n.d. "CrossFit Workouts: It's Time We Stop Glorifying the 'pain cave.'" *Well+Good*. Accessed August 20, 2022. www.wellandgood.com.
Kerry, Victoria J. 2016. "The Construction of Hegemonic Masculinity in the Semiotic Landscape of a CrossFit 'Cave.'" *Visual Communication* 16 (2): 209–237.
King, Tiffany Lethabo, Jenell Navarro, and Andrea Smith, eds. 2020. *Otherwise Worlds: Against Settler Colonialism and Anti-Blackness*. Durham, NC: Duke University Press.
Kivel, Paul. 2013. *Living in the Shadow of the Cross: Understanding and Resisting the Power and Privilege of Christian Hegemony*. Gabriola Island, BC: New Society.
Klippenstein, Kristian. 2013. "Peoples Temple as Christian History: A Corrective Interpretation." In *Alternative Considerations of Jonestown and Peoples Temple*. San Diego: San Diego State University, July 25, 2013. https://jonestown.sdsu.edu.

Knapp, Bobbi A. 2015a. "Gender Representation in the CrossFit Journal: A Content Analysis." *Sport in Society* 18 (6): 688–703.

———. 2015b. "Rx'd and Shirtless: An Examination of Gender in a CrossFit Box." *Women in Sport and Physical Activity Journal* 23 (1): 42–53.

Kupper, Crystal. 2023. "CrossFit for Duty: Soldiers Lean on Functional Fitness to Stay in Shape." *Reserve + National Guard*, March 27, 2023. https://reservenationalguard.com.

Ladd, Tony, and James A. Mathisen. 1999. *Muscular Christianity: Evangelical Protestantism and the Development of American Sport*. Grand Rapids, MI: Baker Books.

Ladd-Taylor, Molly. n.d. "Fitter Family Contests." Eugenics Archives. Accessed July 5, 2024. www.eugenicsarchive.ca.

Lange, Maggie. 2021. "Why Is Talking about Exercise So Uncomfortable?" *The Cut*, September 3, 2021. www.thecut.com.

Latour, Bruno. 1988. *Science in Action: How to Follow Scientists and Engineers through Society*. Cambridge, MA: Harvard University Press.

Lawrence, John Shelton, and Robert Jewett 2002. *The Myth of the American Superhero*. Grand Rapids, MI: William B. Eerdmans.

Learned Handle. 2017. "Strong People Are Harder to Kill (survival story from this weekend)." r/CrossFit, Reddit. www.reddit.com.

Lelwica, Michelle Mary. 2017. *Shameful Bodies: Religion and the Culture of Physical Improvement*. New York: Bloomsbury.

Lemay, Eric. 2013. "CrossFit Mirrors American Militarism." *Salon*, September 8, 2013. www.salon.com.

Lemmon, Gayle Tzemach. 2017. "No Turning Back? First Woman Makes Army's Elite 75th Ranger Regiment, Big Step for Women in Combat." *Defense One*, January 19, 2017. www.defenseone.com.

Library of Congress. n.d. *Classroom Materials: Westward Expansion: Encounters at a Cultural Crossroads*. Accessed July 5, 2024. www.loc.gov.

Lofranco, Justin. 2020. "CrossFit Cancels Athletes Unleashed's Affiliation after Derogatory Email." *Morning Chalk Up*, November 28, 2020. https://morningchalkup.com.

Lofton, Kathryn. 2006. "Practicing Oprah; or, the Prescriptive Compulsion of a Spiritual Capitalism." *Journal of Popular Culture* 39 (4): 599–621.

———. 2011. *Oprah: The Gospel of an Icon*. Chicago: University of Chicago Press.

———. 2017. *Consuming Religion*. Chicago: University of Chicago Press.

Lundskow, George. 2022. "Conspiracies and Restorative Violence in American Culture." *Critical Sociology* 48 (6): 967–987.

Luther, Claudia. 2011. "Jack LeLanne Dies at 96: Spiritual Father of U.S. Fitness Movement." *Los Angeles Times*, January 23, 2011. www.latimes.com.

Macfadden, Bernarr, and Felix Oswald. 1903. *Fasting—Hydropathy—Exercise: Nature's Wonderful Remedies for the Cure of All Chronic and Acute Diseases*. London: Bernarr Macfadden.

MacIntyre, Alasdair. 2007. *After Virtue*. 3rd ed. South Bend, IN: University of Notre Dame Press.

Maguire, Jennifer Smith. 2008. "Leisure and the Obligation of Self-Work: An Examination of the Fitness Field." *Leisure Studies* 27 (1): 59–75.
Markschies, Christoph. 2007. "Der Schmerz und das Christentum. Symbol für Schmerzbewältigung?" [Pain and Christianity. A Symbol for Overcoming Pain?]. *Schmerz* 4:347–350.
Marquez, Tommy. 2020. "Watch: Former CrossFit Employee, Pilot to Greg Glassman Speaks Out." *Morning Chalk Up*, June 12, 2020. https://morningchalkup.com.
Masco, Joseph. 2014. *The Theater of Operations: National Security Affect from the Cold War to the War on Terror*. Durham, NC: Duke University Press.
Mastrorillo, Alessia. 2023. "Between My Breaths: CrossFit as a Depathologizing Healing Strategy for Sexual Trauma Survivors." In *Gender and Power in Strength Sports: Strong as Feminist*, Critical Studies in Sport Series, edited by Noelle K. Brigden, Katie Rose Hejtmanek, and Melissa M. Forbis, 174–191. Abingdon, UK: Routledge.
Mauss, Marcel. 1973. "Techniques of the Body." *Economy and Society* (2) 1: 70–88.
McAdams, Dan. 2006. *The Redemptive Self: Stories Americans Live By*. Oxford: Oxford University Press.
———. 2008. "American Identity: The Redemptive Self." *General Psychologist* 43 (1): 20–27.
McCloud, Sean. 2004. *Making the American Religious Fringe: Exotics, Subversives, and Journalists, 1955–1993*. Chapel Hill: University of North Carolina Press.
McKenzie, Shelly. 2013. *Getting Physical: The Rise of Fitness Culture in America*. Lawrence: University Press of Kansas.
McNulty, Rose. n.d. "The Badass Real Women Playing Amazons in 'Wonder Woman.'" *Muscle and Fitness*. Accessed December 12, 2023. www.muscleandfitness.com.
Mead, Margaret. 1928. *Coming of Age in Samoa*. New York: HarperCollins.
Meador, Keith G. 2003. "'My Own Salvation': The Christian Century and Psychology's Secularization of American Protestantism." In *The Secular Revolution: Power, Interests, and Conflict in the Secularization of American Public Life*, edited by Christian Smith, 269–309. Berkeley: University of California Press.
Meenan, Devin. 2022. "The 10 Years with the Most Superhero Movie Releases, Ranked." *CBR*, January 2, 2022. www.cbr.com.
Merritt, Greg. 2022. "The Power of Positive Thinking." *The Barbell*, October 10, 2022. https://thebarbell.com.
Merry, Sally Engle. 2011. "Measuring the World: Indicators, Human Rights, and Global Governance." *Current Anthropology* 52 (S3): S83–S95.
Mestel, Spenser. 2020. "CrossFit Is Feeling the Weight of Gym Owners Downplaying COVID-19." *BuzzFeed News*, December 23, 2020. www.buzzfeednews.com.
Michelutti, Lucia. 2010. "Wrestling with (Body) Politics: Understanding 'Goonda' Political Styles in North India." In *Power and Influence in India: Bosses, Lords, and Captains*, edited by Pamela Price and Arild Engelsen Ruud, 44–69. New Delhi: Routledge India.
Mills, Anthony R. 2014. *American Theology, Superhero Comics, and Cinema: The Marvel of Stan Lee and the Revolution of a Genre*. New York: Routledge.

Moore, R. Laurence. 2003. *Touchdown Jesus: The Mixing of Sacred and Secular in American History*. Louisville, KY: Westminster John Knox Press.

Morrison, Toni. 1992. *Playing in the Dark: Whiteness and the Literary Imagination*. Cambridge, MA: Harvard University Press.

Murphy, T. J. 2012. *Inside the Box: How CrossFit® Shredded Rules, Stripped Down the Gym, and Rebuilt My Body*. Boulder, CO: Velo.

Musselman, Cody. 2019. "Training for the 'Unknown and Unknowable': CrossFit and Evangelical Temporality." *Religions* 10 (11): 624–643.

———. 2020. "Survival of the CrossFittest: After a Schism over Racism Can the Fitness Empire Shed Its Culture of Whiteness?" *Religion Dispatches*, October 22, 2020. https://religiondispatches.org.

———. 2022. "'Be More Human': CrossFit, Reebok, and Sporting Consumerism." In *Religion and Sport in North America*, edited by Jeffrey Scholes and Randal Balmer, 162–181. New York: Routledge.

———. 2024. "Drinking the CrossFit Kool-Aid: Cult Marketing Meets Functional Fitness." In *Selling the Sacred: Religion and Marketing from CrossFit to QAnon*, edited by Mara Einstein and Sarah MacFarland Taylor, 233–249. New York: Routledge.

National Guard. n.d. *The Rough Riders*. Accessed July 5, 2024. www.nationalguard.mil.

Nuñez, Kristen. 2020. "What Is a 'Pain Cave' and How Do You Power through It in a Workout or Race?" *Healthline*, June 15, 2020. www.healthline.com.

Ocobock, Cara. 2023. "Be Careful, If You Lift Too Heavy Your Boobs Will Shrink." In *Gender and Power in Strength Sports: Strong as Feminist*, Critical Studies in Sport Series, edited by Noelle K. Brigden, Katie Rose Hejtmanek, and Melissa M. Forbis, 143–148. Abingdon, UK: Routledge.

Ocobock, Cara, and Katie Rose Hejtmanek. 2022. "Missing the Gym: COVID-19 Stay-at-Home Orders and Formal Fitness Communities." *Anthropology Now* 14 (1–2): 112–116.

———. 2023. "'I Exercise with Others in about 6–7 Online Fitness Communities': Women's Exercise Routine and Resilience during COVID-19 Stay at Home Orders." In *Gender and Power in Strength Sports: Strong as Feminist*, Critical Studies in Sport Series, edited by Noelle K. Brigden, Katie Rose Hejtmanek, and Melissa M. Forbis, 192–214. Abingdon, UK: Routledge.

Ocobock, Cara, Sarah Lacy, and Alexandra Niclou. 2021. "Between a Rock and a Cold Place: Neanderthal Biocultural Cold Adaptations." *Evolutionary Anthropology* 30:262–279.

Ojimba, Anthony C., and Bruno Yammeluan. 2019. "Friedrich Nietzsche's Superman and Its Religious Implications." *Journal of Philosophy, Culture and Religion* 45:17–25.

Oldenburg, Ray. 1989. *The Great Good Place: Cafes, Coffee Shops, Community Centers, Beauty Parlors, General Stores, Bars, Hangouts, and How They Get You through the Day*. New York: Paragon House.

One Church. 2013. "One Church | CrossFit New Albany Campus." YouTube, September 6, 2013. www.youtube.com/watch?v=GRRPTmm-HmY.

Ornella, Alexander D. 2015. "Clothed with Strength: Meaningful Material Practices in the Sport of CrossFit." *The Jugaad Project: Material Religions in Context* (blog), August 9, 2015. www.thejugaadproject.pub.

———. 2019. "'Jesus Saves' and 'Clothed in Christ': Athletic Religious Apparel in the Christian CrossFit Community." *Sport in Society* 22 (2): 266–280.

Osorio, David. 2014. "Why Are CrossFit Gyms so Expensive?" *Inside the Affiliate* (blog), December 22, 2014. www.insidetheaffiliate.com.

O'Sullivan, John. 1839. "The Divine Destiny of America." *New Humanist* www.newhumanist.com.

Palahniuk, Chuck. 1996. *Fight Club*. New York: Norton.

Pavlidis, Adele, and Simone Fullagar. 2015. "The Pain and Pleasure of Roller Derby: Thinking through Affect and Subjectification." *International Journal of Cultural Studies* 18 (5): 483–499.

Peale, Norman Vincent. 1952. *The Power of Positive Thinking*. New York: Prentice Hall.

Peck, Janice. 2008. *The Age of Oprah: Cultural Icon for the Neoliberal Era*. Boulder, CO: Paradigm.

———. 2010. "The Secret of Her Success: Oprah Winfrey and the Seductions of Self-Transformation." *Journal of Communication Inquiry* 34 (1): 7–14.

Perkins, Judith. 1995. *The Suffering Self: Pain and Narrative Representation in the Early Christian Era*. London: Routledge.

Petrzela, Natalia Mehlman. 2016. "When Wellness Is a Dirty Word." *Chronicle of Higher Education*, May 1, 2016. www.chronicle.com.

———. 2022. *Fit Nation: The Gains and Pains of America's Exercise Obsession*. Chicago: University of Chicago Press.

Pettersen, Susan Dahl, Per M. Aslaksen, and Svein Arne Pettersen. 2020. "Pain Processing in Elite and High-Level Athletes Compared to Non-athletes." *Frontiers in Psychology* 11:1908.

Pew Research Center. 2014. "Religious Landscape Study." www.pewresearch.org.

Pickett, Andrew C., Andrew Goldsmith, Zack Damon, and Matthew Walker. 2016. "The Influence of Sense of Community on the Perceived Value of Physical Activity: A Cross-Context Analysis." *Leisure Sciences* 38 (3): 199–214.

Pipes, Tim. 2016. "Defense Never Rests." *CrossFit Journal*, January 9, 2016. http://library.crossfit.com.

Pobiner, Briana. 2018. "What Can Fossils Tell Us about Early Human Diets?" *Anthropology News*, October 17, 2018.

Power, Michael. 1994. *The Audit Explosion*. London: Demos.

———. 1996. "Making Things Auditable." *Accounting, Organizations and Society* 2 (2–3): 289–315.

———. 1999. *The Audit Society: Rituals of Verification*. Oxford: Oxford University Press.

Powers, Devon, and D. M. Greenwell. 2017. "Branded Fitness: Exercise and Promotional Culture." *Journal of Consumer Culture* 17 (3): 523–541.

Preston, Andrew. 2012. *Sword of the Spirit, Shield of Faith: Religion in American War and Diplomacy*. New York: Penguin Random House.

Pronger, Brian. 2002. *Body Fascism: Salvation in the Technology of Physical Fitness.* Toronto: University of Toronto Press.

Putney, Clifford. 2001. *Muscular Christianity: Manhood and Sports in Protestant American, 1880–1920.* Cambridge, MA: Harvard University Press.

Rally Fitness. 2017. "The Business of CrossFit: An Update on New Market Research." March 13, 2017. https://rallyfitness.com.

Rapisarda, Eric. 2020. "Chalk Talk: Recording Your Score." Daybreak CrossFit, February 17, 2020. https://daybreakcrossfit.com.

Raynsford, Jody. 2021. *How to Start a Cult: Be Bold, Build Belonging, and Attract a Band of Devoted Followers to Your Brand.* Monee, IL: Known Publishing.

r/CrossFit. 2019. "Why Do Some Consider CrossFit a Cult?" Reddit, June 4, 2019. www.reddit.com.

ReasonTV. 2013. "CrossFit Founder Greg Glassman: 'I'm a Rabid Libertarian.'" YouTube, July 22, 2013. www.youtube.com/watch?v=-EB0XyBUl0U.

Redwood-Brown, Athalie. 2022. "Impact on Habitual CrossFit Participant's Exercise Behavior, Health, and Well-Being: A Cross-Sectional Survey of UK COVID-19 Lockdowns." *Health Science Reports* 6:e1140.

Retraction Watch. 2017. "Ohio State Exercise Researcher Resigns after Retraction of CrossFit Study." *Retractionwatch.com*, June 12, 2017. https://retractionwatch.com.

Reynolds, Lucas. 2022. "Why Is CrossFit So Expensive? (11 Reasons Why)." *VeryInformed*, June 14, 2022. https://veryinformed.com.

Roanhorse, Rebecca. 2018. *The Trail of Lightning.* New York: Saga.

Rodgers, Daniel. T. 2018. *As a City on a Hill: The Story of America's Most Famous Lay Sermon.* Princeton, NJ: Princeton University Press.

Rogers, Jeffrey. 2023. "Average Navy SEAL Height According 2023." *From Military Bases*, January 2, 2023. https://frommilitarybases.com.

Rogue Fitness. n.d. "The Rogue Way: About Us." Accessed July 8, 2024. www.roguefitness.com.

Rosman, Katherine. 2020a. "CrossFit Owner Fostered Sexist Company Culture, Workers Say." *New York Times*, June 20, 2020. www.nytimes.com.

———. 2020b. "Greg Glassman, Embattled Owner of CrossFit, to Sell His Company." *New York Times*, June 24, 2020. www.nytimes.com.

Rossillo, Amanda. 2022. "How Our Evolutionary Past Shapes Our Health Today." *American Scientist*, February 25, 2022. www.americanscientist.org.

Royce, Josiah. 1886. *California: A Study of American Character: From the Conquest in 1846 to the Second Vigilance Committee in San Francisco.* Boston: Houghton Mifflin.

———. 1899. *The World and the Individual: The Gifford Lectures.* New York: Macmillan.

———. (1913) 1968. *The Problem of Christianity.* Gateway ed. 2 vols. Chicago: Henry Regnery.

Royce, Sarah. 1932. *A Frontier Lady: Recollections of the Gold Rush and Early California.* New Haven, CT: Yale University Press.

Royse, Alyssa. 2020. "CrossFit, Black Lives and Covid." Rocket Community Fitness, June 5, 2020. www.rocketcommunityfitness.com.

Sarason, Seymour B. 1974. *The Psychological Sense of Community: Prospects for a Community Psychology.* San Francisco: Jossey-Bass.

Scarry, Elaine. 1985. *The Body in Pain: The Making and Unmaking of the World.* Oxford: Oxford University Press.

Schulson, Michael. 2017. "Is American Christianity Becoming a Workout Cult?" *The Daily Beast*, July 12, 2017. www.thedailybeast.com.

Schwartz, Roy. 2022. "Men of Steel: Superman vs Übermensch." *Philosophy Now* 148. https://philosophynow.org.

Sen, Sohini. 2023. "Bulky Is Not the Worst Thing a Woman Can Be." In *Gender and Power in Strength Sports: Strong as Feminist*, Critical Studies in Sport Series, edited by Noelle K. Brigden, Katie Rose Hejtmanek, and Melissa M. Forbis, 19–26. Abingdon, UK: Routledge.

Sharpe, Christina. 2016. *In the Wake: On Blackness and Being.* Durham, NC: Duke University Press.

Shore, Cris, and Susan Wright. 2015. "Audit Culture: Rankings, Ratings, and the Reassembling of Society." *Current Anthropology* 56 (3): 421–444.

Simpson, Duncan, Tanya R. Prewitt-White, Yuri Feito, Julianne Giusti, and Ryan Shuda. 2017. "Challenge, Commitment, Community, and Empowerment: Factors That Promote the Adoption of CrossFit as a Training Regimen." *Sport Journal*, May 1, 2017. https://thesportjournal.org.

Slatta, Richard W. 2001. *The Mythical West: An Encyclopedia of Legend, Lore, and Popular Culture.* Santa Barbara, CA: ABC-CLIO.

Slotkin, Richard. 1973. *Regeneration through Violence: The Mythology of the American Frontier, 1600–1860.* Middleton, CT: Wesleyan University Press.

———. 1985. *The Fatal Environment: The Myth of the Frontier in the Age of Industrialization, 1800–1890.* New York: Atheneum.

———. 1998. *Gunfighter Nation: The Myth of the Frontier in Twentieth-Century America.* Norman: University of Oklahoma Press.

Smith, Christian. 2003. "Introduction: Rethinking the Secularization of American Public Life." In *The Secular Revolution: Power, Interests, and Conflict in the Secularization of American Life*, edited by Christian Smith, 1–96. Berkeley: University of California Press.

Smith, Martin Cruz. (1970) 1981. *The Indians Won.* 2nd ed. New York: Leisure Press.

Spencer, Dale C. 2009. "Habit(Us), Body Techniques and Body Callusing: An Ethnography of Mixed Martial Arts." *Body & Society* 15 (4): 119–143.

Spielvogel, Laura. 2003. *Working Out in Japan: Shaping the Female Body in Tokyo Fitness Clubs.* Durham, NC: Duke University Press.

Spry, Adam. 2020. "Decolonial Eschatologies of Native American Literatures." In *Apocalypse in American Literature and Culture*, edited by John Hay, 55–67. Cambridge: Cambridge University Press.

Starker, Steven. (1989) 2008. *Oracle at the Supermarket: The American Preoccupation with Self-Help Books.* New Brunswick, NJ: Transaction.

Stone, Livia K. Under review. *Autogestión in Motion: Popularizing Anarchist Ethics from Algerian Revolution to Mexico City Punk.* Durham, NC: Duke University Press.

Strathern, Marilyn. 1996–1967. "From Improvement to Enhancement: An Anthropological Comment on the Audit Culture." *Cambridge Journal of Anthropology* 19 (3): 1–21.
Strauss, Sara. 2005. *Positioning Yoga: Balancing Acts across Cultures*. New York: Berg.
Strumpf, Andy. 2020. "Full Auto Friday—Round 5." *Cleared Hot Podcast*, YouTube, June 12, 2020. www.youtube.com/watch?v=tTxzym5KHjQ.
Sutton, Matthew Avery. 2014. *American Apocalypse: A History of Modern Evangelicalism*. Cambridge, MA: Harvard University Press.
Ta, Lynn M. 2006. "Hurt So Good: *Fight Club*, Masculine Violence, and the Crisis of Capitalism." *Journal of American Culture* 29 (3): 265–277.
Tao, David. 2023. "Rich Froning Releases Statement on Greg Glassman Twitter Controversy." *BarBend*, updated July 31, 2023. https://barbend.com. The original Froning statement was on June 7, 2020, on Instagram.
Taylor, Frederick Winslow. (1913) 1997. *The Principles of Scientific Management*. Mineola, NY: Dover.
Thurston, Angie, and Casper ter Kuile. 2015. *How We Gather—A New Report on Nonreligious Community*. Cambridge, MA: Harvard Divinity School. https://caspertk.files.wordpress.com.
TimWaltonTV. 2020. "Buffalo, New York Business Owners Stand Up to Cuomo Lockdown Orders: Chase Out Sheriff & Health Dept." YouTube, November 20, 2020. www.youtube.com/watch?v=AI_pkvlp2q4.
Tocqueville, Alexis de. 1838. *1805–1859. Democracy in America*. New York: G. Dearborn.
Trujillo, Nick. 1991. "Hegemonic Masculinity on the Mound: Media representations of Nolan Ryan and American Sports Culture." *Critical Studies in Media Communications* 8:290–308.
Turner, Edith. 2011. *Communitas: The Anthropology of Collective Joy*. New York: Palgrave Macmillan.
Turner, Victor. 1967. *The Forest of Symbols: Aspects of Ndembu Ritual*. Ithaca, NY: Cornell University Press.
———. 1969. *The Ritual Process: Structure and Anti-Structure*. Chicago: Aldine.
Turtiainen, Riika, and Usva Friman. 2023. "Strength over Gender? Discussing and Presenting the Ambivalent Female Strength in the CrossFit Games 2019." In *Gender and Power in Strength Sports: Strong as Feminist*, Critical Studies in Sport Series, edited by Noelle K. Brigden, Katie Rose Hejtmanek, and Melissa M. Forbis, 29–53. Abingdon, UK: Routledge.
Tuveson, Ernest Lee. 1968. *Redeemer Nation: The Idea of America's Millennial Role*. Chicago: University of Chicago Press.
Ulrich, Madeline. 2016. "Why CrossFitters Talk about CrossFit So Much: The Fittest on Earth." *The Odyssey Online, Health and Wellness*, July 18, 2016. www.theodysseyonline.com.
Ultimate Performance. 2021. "The Power of Positive Thinking." *Ultimate Performance* (blog), July 1, 2021. https://blog.ultimateperformance.com.
Vennare, Anthony. n.d. "Rogue's Under-the-Radar Dominance." *Fitt Insider*. Accessed July 5, 2024. https://insider.fitt.co.

Wagner, Rachel. 2025. *Cowboy Apocalypse: Religion, Media, Guns*. New York: New York University Press.
Waller, David. 2011. *The Perfect Man: The Muscular Life and Times of Eugene Sandow Victorian Strongman*. Brighton, UK: Victorian Secrets Limited.
Walsh, John. 2006. "Could It Be Cult Fitness?" *CrossFit Discussion Board*, December 20, 2006. https://board.crossfit.com.
Washington, Myra S., and Megan Economides. 2016. "Strong Is the New Sexy: Women, CrossFit, and the Postfeminist Ideal." *Journal of Sport and Social Issues* 40 (2): 143–161.
Weber, Max. 1930. *The Protestant Ethic and the Spirit of Capitalism*. London: George Allen and Unwin.
Wertsch, James V. 2019. *How Nations Remember: A Narrative Approach*. Oxford: Oxford University Press.
Wessinger Catherine. 2009. "'Cults' in America: Discourse and Outcomes." In *The Cambridge History of Religions in America*, edited by Stephen J. Stein, 511–531. Cambridge: Cambridge University Press.
Wiese, Kay. 2023. "Kettle Wedding Bells: CrossFit 1886 Pulls Off Gym Wedding on One Day's Notice." *Morning Chalk Up*, August 30, 2023. https://morningchalkup.com.
Wise, Damon. 2000. "Now You See It . . ." *The Guardian*, November 2, 2000. www.theguardian.com.
WNYMedia Network. 2020. "Athletes Unleashed Owner Sends Racist Vile Response to Buffalo Woman Asking for a Refund." *WNYMedia.net*, November 25, 2020. https://wnymedia.net.
Wolf, Daniel R. 1991. *The Rebels: A Brotherhood of Outlaw Bikers*. Toronto: University of Toronto Press.
Wolf, Robb. n.d. "What Is the Paleo Diet?" Robb Wolf's website. Accessed July 5, 2024. https://robbwolf.com.
World Population Review. 2023. "Average Height by State 2023." https://worldpopulationreview.com.
Youngs, J. William T. 1998. *The Congregationalists*. New York: Bloomsbury.

INDEX

affiliates, CrossFit, 6, 30, 67; annual fee due to CrossFit HQ, 177; as antifranchise, 62; congregationalist churches and, 68; CrossFit gyms as, 68, 103; frontier and, 82; sacred covenant with, 61, 62

afterlives: American historical, 5; Christianity, 5, 28, 155, 175, 176, 185n15; settler Christian colonialism, 8, 178

Alfonsi, Sharyn, 1–2, 5–6, 103

American Christianity: American myth and, 16; culture and, 29; decline of, 17; frontier and, 83; hero myths and, 112; history, 4–5; self-help and, 63, 64, 65–66; society and, 16, 17; superheroes and, 113

American culture, 5; apocalypse and, 18–19, 152–56; Christianity and, 29; frontier myth and, 87, 89; garage in, 70–71, 73; violence and, 93, 94. *See also* American popular culture

American frontier. *See* frontier, American

American history: apocalypse and, 152–53; Christianity in, 4–5; CrossFit and afterlives of, 5. *See also* frontier, American

American institutions, secularism of, 17

American myth: Christianity and, 16; garage and, 73; hero monomyth, 106, 107–8, 112, 115, 124. *See also* frontier myth

American narratives, 7, 50–52

American popular culture, 108; end times in, 152–56; religion and, 16, 24–25; research of, 15–16; superhero monomyth in, 108

American Protestantism, 64, 65, 153, 197n8

Americans: Christians and, 113; self of, 50, 52; whiteness and, 113

American society: Christianity and, 16, 17; frontier myth and, 87; quantification of daily life, 131–32

American stories: Christian stories and, 51; NNPs, 7, 99; redemption stories, 49–50, 52; salvation stories, 49, 50

American themes, in CrossFit stories, 7

America's wake, 4, 13, 16, 185n12

AMRAP workouts, 183, 195n2

Amundson, Greg, 90

anthropology: CrossFit workouts and, 8–15, 186n18; definitions of community in, 33; on diet, 143–45; psychology and, 51, 191n34; of science, 149

apocalypse: American culture and, 18–19, 152–56; American history and, 152–53; Christianity and, 152–55; CrossFit and, 18–19, 151–52, 155–56, 164, 167, 178; end times and, 153; Indigenous people and, 155; racialized Christian stories about, 155, 197n16, 197n18; white evangelicals and, 154–55, 197n18; white male elites and, 151; zombie, 28, 151, 152, 155, 188n45

Aristotelian model of science, 130–31, 132

Asad, Talal, 185n15, 191n35

Atkin, Douglas, 75

audit culture, 132–33, 137, 139–41

audit systems, 132

Augustine, 40

Australia CrossFit, 173
Authentic Fakes (Chidester), 15, 24

Bacon, Francis, 131, 132, 148
Beckwith, Michael, 66
beloved community, 34–35, 37–38, 69, 168
benchmark workouts, 121–22
Berger, Russell, 146
Beyond the Whiteboard (BTWB), 129
big-box gym, 74
Billington, Ray, 85, 86
Black, Jonathan, 26
Black Lives Matter, 156–57, 159
Black people: apocalypse stories and, 155; CrossFit and, 161–63; Glassman, CrossFit and, 156–62. *See also* race
body, CrossFit: of CrossFit Games athletes, 111–12; CrossFit heroes and, 110, 121; Glassman's body and, 123; whiteness of, 112, 113; of women, 119, 121
body fascism, 149
boxes, CrossFit, 2, 6, 183; as garage gyms, 74, 75; Glassman's first, 59, 62; identity and, 30; local community and, 69; as pilgrimage sites, 69. *See also* gyms, CrossFit
Brand, Dionne, 4
brands: CrossFit, 62, 70, 74; cult, 30; Winfrey as, 66
BTWB. *See* Beyond the Whiteboard
burpees (exercise), 46, 183

Campbell, Joseph, 107
capitalism, collectivism vs., 178
capitalism, CrossFit and: different forms of, 62; garage, 63, 73, 75; oracle capitalism of, 62–63
Castro, Dave, 90, 161, 172, 194n42; CrossFit Games and, 91, 101, 110
Catholicism, 191n33
Cavill, Henry, 111
Chidester, David, 15, 24
Christian community, 46, 52–53

Christianity: afterlives, 5, 28, 155, 175, 176, 185n15; apocalypse and, 152–55; book of Jonah, 190n25; "Drinking the Kool-Aid" and, 22; end times, 153–55, 197n16; fitness and, 25–29; hierarchical systems of, 68; imperialism and, 8, 94, 95, 148; Muscular Christianity, 27; narratives of, 50–52; pain and suffering in, 45–46, 48, 49, 52, 189n8; racialized apocalypse stories and, 155, 197n16, 197n18; science and, 148; Second Coming of Jesus and rapture in, 153–55; US's foundation and, 16–17, 185n16; white evangelical apocalypticism, 154–55, 197n18; whiteness and, 113. *See also* cultural Christianity
Christianity, CrossFit and, 3, 23–24, 37; cultural, 5, 17, 18, 29, 52; gyms and, 27–28, 69; pain and, 47–49, 52, 190n27
Christianity's wake, 178; CrossFit and, 3, 15, 17, 28–29, 175; of settler Christian colonialism, 176
Christians: Americans and, 113; American stories and stories of, 51; imperialism of white male, 8, 94; white heteronormative, 113
CK. *See* CrossFit Kids
coaches, CrossFit, 67, 68, 90, 104, 125–27
collectivism, 178
community: American frontier, 85–86, 193n10; anthropological definitions of, 33; beloved, 34–35, 37–38, 69, 168; boxes and local, 69; Christian, 46, 52–53; millennials and, 33; romance of, 168
community, CrossFit, 33, 44; "agony and laughter" of, 35, 36; alchemic process of, 32; as beloved community, 34–35, 37–38, 69, 168; as branded, 62; CVFM@HI + Communal Environment = Health, 31–32; Glassman on, 33, 103; as greatest contribution, 140; growth of, 62; gym, 114; as local and global, 68–69; masculinity and, 35–37;

pain and salvation in, 57–58; sense of, 32
community identity: Christian, 46, 52–53; CrossFit, 35, 168
competitions, CrossFit, 198n1; "Friday Night Lights," 12; international, 3, 171. *See also* CrossFit Games
Confessions (Augustine), 40, 41
congregationalist churches, 68
Cooperman, Stephanie, 22
COVID-19 pandemic: apocalypse, CrossFitters and, 19, 155–56, 164, 167; CrossFitters and, 19, 155–56, 164–68; fracturing of CrossFit and, 168; Glassman and, 155–59, 166, 167; stay-at-home orders and, 164–68; survey, 165
Crockett, Davy, 88
CrossFit, 183; American themes in stories of, 7; appeal, 3; audit culture and, 133, 137, 139–41; autogestión, 177; blog, 127; business model, 59–62, 78; classes, 125–26; conventionality of, 175; culture, 162, 163; ethos, 91; excellence valued over money, 61; as expensive, 14; as fantasy, 175–76; financial success, 6, 60–61; future, 169, 178; garage and, 69–76; legacy, 176; libertarianism in ethos of, 91; life changes due to, 104–6; mascots, 36, 55–56; media, 14; moral authority, 61, 62, 67; narrative templates, 7–8; newer mature version, 174–75; NNPs, 7, 8; popularity in US, 2, 3; practice, 12; self-improvement and, 3; shoes, 21; stories, 5, 7–8; virtuous life and, 17–18, 187n46. *See also specific topics*
CrossFit Defense, 100
CrossFit definitions: CVFM@HI + Communal Environment = Health, 31–32; "Defining CrossFit" video, 135–37; fitness in, 133–41, 146; in 100 Words, 139–40; science and, 135–37, 140
CrossFit Games, 3, 103, 136, 169; appearance of athletes, 111–12; Castro and, 91, 101, 110; finals (2015), 1; first round, 12; "Fittest on Earth," 101, 110–12, 194n42; heroism of athletes, 110; white people in, 163; women in, 116, 119, 120
CrossFit Health, 147, 149
CrossFit HQ, 61, 159, 172, 174, 177; sexism of Glassman and, 160–61, 167, 168
CrossFit Journal, 59, 61, 67, 72, 74, 103; "What Is Fitness?," 137–38; Ziniewicz story in, 114–15
CrossFit Kids (CK), 48–49
CrossFit Open, 12, 110–11
CrossFit Ranch, 91
CrossFitters: American themes in stories of, 7; apocalypse, COVID-19 and, 19, 155–56, 164, 167; COVID-19 pandemic and, 19, 155–56, 164–68; demographics, 13–14; disaffiliation from CrossFit of, 160; as elite, 14; in film, 111; as heroes, 110, 117–19, 124; identity, 35, 36, 37; individualism, 177–78; as proselytizers, 24; from US military, 97; whiteness of, 14, 37; zombie apocalypse preparation by, 155. *See also* body, CrossFit; women CrossFitters
CrossFitting, communication of, 11–12
cult, CrossFit as, 2, 3, 18, 29, 37; "Drinking the Kool-Aid" and, 21–23; Glassman and, 21–23, 30, 31; as good cult, 22; Musselman on, 30, 31
The Culting of Brands (Atkin), 75
cults: cult brands, 30; "Drinking the Kool-Aid" in, 21–22; Musselman on, 29, 30; religion and, 29–30
cultural Christianity, 4, 176; American psychology and, 51; CrossFit and, 5, 17, 18, 29, 52; racialized apocalypse stories and, 155, 197n16, 197n18; redemption stories and, 52; self-help books and, 65–66; wake of, 178
culture: audit, 132–33, 137, 139–41; embodiment of, 11; fitness, 26; science and, 149. *See also* American culture

Curves, 74
CVFM@HI (constantly varied functional movement at high intensity), 31–32
CVFM@HI + Communal Environment = Health, 31–32

Dalton, Francis, 145
Darby, John Nelson, 153
Dawson, Marcelle, 3, 187n46
deadlift, 125–27
"Defining CrossFit" video, 135–37
delayed-onset muscle soreness (DOMS), 56
diet: anthropology on, 143–45; CrossFit, 2, 106; paleo, 2, 130, 142–43, 144
DOMS. *See* delayed-onset muscle soreness
double-unders, 183
dropped in (stopping at local CrossFit gyms), 11

Easter, Michael, 147
end times: in American popular culture, 152–56; apocalypse and, 153; Christianity and, 153–55, 197n16; collectivism and, 178; CrossFit and, 151–52, 177; postmillennialism, 153–54, 197n8; premillennialism, 153–55, 197n8. *See also* apocalypse
ergs (rowing machines), 150
Erlanger, Olivia, 70, 73, 75
ESPN, 1
eugenics, 113, 145
evangelicals, apocalypticism of white, 154–55, 197n18
Every Second Counts, 119
evolutionary science, 141–46

FAITH RXD, 27–28
Farnell, Brenda, 11
femininity, heteronormative, 119–20, 122
Fight Club (Palahniuk), 36–37
fitness: body fascism and, 149; Christianity and, 25–29; culture, 26; functional, 31–32, 130, 141, 142; industry, 148; religion and, 26–27; science and, 133; survival of fittest, 145–46; trends in India 2018, 172–73
fitness, CrossFit and, 10, 27, 186n19; definitions of, 133–41, 146; functional, 31–32, 130, 141, 142; Glassman on, 67, 133–37, 146, 164; standards of, 137–39; US military and, 63, 78–80, 90–91, 96–97, 100, 101; work capacity in, 133–34, 135
Floyd, George, 156–57, 159, 161, 162, 168
Fluffy Duck meme, 166
Ford, Henry, 132
Fran, 10, 56, 183
"Friday Night Lights" competition, 12
Friman, Usva, 120
Froning, Rich, 1, 27, 111, 160, 188n39, 196n31
frontier, American: American identity and, 86, 87; Christianity and, 83; community of, 85–86, 193n10; heroes of, 86–89, 106; Indigenous people and, 84–86, 94, 193n5, 193n8, 193n10; settler Christian colonialism, 8, 50, 82, 85, 86, 87, 93–95, 176, 178; settler-rangers and militias, 88, 193n14; survival of fittest in, 145; US military and, 82–83, 91, 96; violence and, 82–84, 86–87, 89, 93–95, 192n1; white males and, 83, 84, 91, 93, 193n5; women and, 122. *See also* frontier myth
frontier, CrossFit and, 101, 175; CrossFit gyms and, 82, 83, 89, 91–93, 102; frontier myth and, 90, 102; Glassman and, 82, 89, 90; hunter-heroes and, 91; overview, 82; US military and, 82–83, 91, 102; Wild West and, 82, 83
frontier line, 84, 85, 86
frontier myth, 83, 85, 193n8; American culture and, 87, 89; American society and, 87; CrossFit and, 90, 102; garage and, 82; hunter myth, 86–87; violence and, 93–94

INDEX | 221

functional fitness, 31–32, 130, 141, 142
functional movements, CrossFit, 141, 142; CVFM@HI, 31–32

garage: American culture and, 70–71, 73; American myth and, 73; CrossFit and, 69–76; frontier myth and, 82; Glassman and, 71–75; heroes of, 71; myth of, 71–74, 82
garage capitalism, 63, 73, 75
garage gyms, CrossFit, 72, 76, 195n1; CrossFit boxes as, 74, 75; garage myth and, 82; overview, 81–82
gear, CrossFit, 59
Geertz, Clifford, 185n16, 191n35
The Girls (benchmark workouts), 10, 121–22, 163, 183
Glassman, Greg, 18; apocalypse, COVID-19 pandemic, CrossFit and, 155–56, 167; audit culture used by, 133, 137; business advice, 59–60, 177; coach training by, 67; COVID-19 pandemic and, 155–59, 166, 167; as creator/designer of CrossFit, 1–2, 5, 67, 90, 123–24, 133, 162, 175; CrossFit as cult and, 21–23, 30, 31; on CrossFit as deadly, 36; CrossFit body and body of, 123; on CrossFit's community, 33, 103; on doing the right thing, 66–67; early life, 73; on evolutionary science and CrossFit, 142; fall of CrossFit and, 155–64, 167–69, 172, 197n24; first CrossFit box, 59, 62; first CrossFit gym opening by, 59, 62; on fitness, 67, 133–37, 146, 164; frontier and, 82, 89, 90; garage and, 71–75; on The Girls, 10, 121, 183; as guru, 61, 62; interviews, 14; lectures, 59–60, 75–76, 134–37; libertarianism of, 6, 82, 89–90, 156, 166, 167; on math and CrossFit, 135–37; moral authority of, 61, 62, 67; NSCA and, 147; race, CrossFit and, 156–62, 167, 168; Roza compared to, 177; sacred covenant with gym owners, 68; on science and CrossFit, 133–37, 142, 146–48, 149, 196n15; sexism of CrossFit HQ and, 160–61, 167, 168; *60 Minutes* interview, 1–2, 5–6; State Policy Network Conference and, 59, 75–76; sugar industry and, 147, 149; US military and, 96–97, 162; videos by, 59, 61, 134–37; vision of, 68–69
Glucklich, Ariel, 45, 52
Govela, Luis Ortega, 70, 73, 75
Green, Marjorie Taylor, 3
Gregory, Sean, 23
Griffith, Marie, 26
Gusterson, Hugh, 149
Guynes, Sean, 108, 112
gym: equipment and Rogue, 76–78; "on and off the bandwagon" narrative, 22
gyms, CrossFit, 9, 125; as affiliates, 68, 103; as anti-gym, 70, 74, 75, 91; Australian, 173; big-box, 74; Christianity and, 27–28, 69; community, 114; COVID-19 stay-at-home orders and, 164–65, 168; disaffiliation of, 159–60, 169; frontier and, 82, 83, 89, 91–93, 102; garage gyms, 72, 74–76, 81–82, 195n1; Glassman's first, 59, 62; Glassman's sacred covenant with owners of, 68; hegemonic masculinity of, 120–21; heroism of, 110, 113–15, 124; international, 15; mainstream gyms compared to, 11, 30, 72, 81, 82, 93; memberships, 14; post COVID-19, 171–72; research on, 146–47; salvation in, 39–44; secularism and, 28; T-shirt, 69; US military and, 91, 97–98; white males and, 70, 80. See also boxes, CrossFit

Hart, Matt, 169, 176
Hartman, Saidiya, 5, 176
Hefferman, Virginia, 23
hegemonic masculinity, CrossFit and, 120–21, 163
Hells Angels, 35–36

heroes: garage, 71; hero's journey, 106, 107; of US military, 89, 95–96; women as, 122
heroes, American: Christianity and myths of, 112; of frontier, 86–89, 106; hunter-heroes, 86–87, 88, 91, 95, 106; monomyth, 106, 107–8, 112, 115, 124; whiteness of, 113. *See also* superheroes, American
heroes, CrossFit, 106; CrossFit body and, 110, 121; CrossFit Game athletes as, 110; CrossFit gym heroism, 110, 113–15, 124; CrossFitters as, 110, 117–19, 124; forms of, 110; women as, 117–18, 122, 124. *See also* Hero WODs; superheroes, CrossFit
Hero WODs, 93, 96, 101, 118–19, 163; CrossFit superheroes and, 16, 106; hunter-heroes and, 106; Murph, 15, 98–100, 183
heteronormative femininity, 119–20, 122
heteronormative whiteness, 112, 113
Heywood, Leslie, 119
hunter-heroes, 86–87, 88, 91, 95, 106

identity: community, 35, 46, 52–53, 168; frontier and American, 86, 87
identity, CrossFit: boxes and, 30; community identity, 35, 168; CrossFitters and, 35, 36, 37; tensions between other identities and, 168
IHME. *See* Institute for Health Metrics and Evaluation
imperialism, Christianity and, 8, 94, 95, 148
Indigenous people: American frontier and, 84–86, 94, 193n5, 193n8, 193n10; apocalypse and, 155; settler Christian colonialism and, 86, 94; whiteness and, 85
Institute for Health Metrics and Evaluation (IHME), 158–59
international, CrossFit, 11, 14; comparison of American and, 173–74; competitions, 3; gyms, 15

Jackson, W. Turrentine, 93
James, William, 51
Jefferson, Thomas, 83, 84
Jewett, Robert, 107, 108, 112
Jonah, 47, 190n25
Jones, Jim, 21–22
Joseph, Miranda, 35, 168
Journal of Strength and Conditioning Research, 146–47
Jung, Carl, 107

Kaepernick, Colin, 156–57
Kerry, Victoria, 120–21
Khalipa, Jason, 119, 160
kip, 10, 173, 183
Kivel, Paul, 17
Knapp, Bobbi, 119

LaLanne, Jack, 26, 27
Latour, Bruno, 148
Lawrence, John Shelton, 107, 108, 112
Lemay, Eric, 70
libertarianism, 6, 82, 89–91, 156, 166, 167
Lofton, Kathryn, 63
Lund, Martin, 108, 112
Lundskow, George, 94, 95

Macfadden, Bernarr, 26, 27
MacIntyre, Alasdaire, 17
Making the American Body (Macfadden and Oswald), 26
Manifest Destiny, 83
Masco, Joseph, 79, 95
masculinity, CrossFit and, 74, 75; CrossFit community and, 35–37; CrossFit workouts and, 36–37; hegemonic, 120–21, 163
math: enumeration, 131, 139; Glassman on CrossFit and, 135–37; Newtonian mechanics and, 134, 136
McAdams, Dan, 49–52
Merry, Sally Engle, 131–32
Mestel, Spencer, 168

MetCon (CrossFit workout metabolic conditioning), 9, 126, 183
millennials, 33
Mills, Anthony, 108
monomyth, American hero, 106, 107–8, 112, 115, 124
Morning Chalk Up, 162, 165
movements: CrossFit, 31–32, 141, 142; human, 141–42
Mulvaney, Brian, 157, 197n24
Murph Hero WOD, 15, 98–100, 183
Murphy, Michael P., 98, 99
Muscular Christianity, 27
Musselman, Cody, 24–25, 113, 145, 150; on CrossFit as cult, 30, 31; on cults, 29, 30

narratives: American, 7, 50–52; Christian, 50–52; CrossFit narrative templates, 7–8; NNPs, 7, 8, 99; "on and off the bandwagon," 22; salvation, 50–52
national narrative projects (NNPs), 7, 8, 99
National Strength and Conditioning Association (NSCA), 133, 146, 147
New Thought, 26–27, 64–65
Newtonian mechanics, 134, 136
New York Times, 22, 55, 160–61
New York Times Magazine, 23
9/11 attacks, 95, 109, 162
NNPs. *See* national narrative projects
NSCA. *See* National Strength and Conditioning Association

Ocobock, Cara, 165
OGs (long-term CrossFit members), 13
oracle, 64; Glassman as, 67; self-help books as, 65, 66; Winfrey as, 65, 66
oracle capitalism, 62–63
Ornella, Alexander, 69
the Other, 94, 95

pain and salvation, CrossFit, 44, 46–47, 52, 53; community and, 57–58

pain and suffering: martyrs and, 189n11; research on, 46, 190n17
pain and suffering, Christian, 48, 189n8; Christian community identity and, 46, 52–53; Christian salvation and, 45–46, 49, 52; community of sufferers, 52–53; suffering self and, 52
pain and suffering, CrossFit: Christianity and, 47–49, 52, 190n27; CrossFit workouts and, 12, 40, 44, 46–49, 54–58; pain cave, 47–49; in WOD, 47, 54–55, 57. *See also* pain and salvation, CrossFit
Palahniuk, Chuck, 36
paleo diet, 2, 130, 142–43, 144
Perkins, Judith, 52
Petrzela, Natalia, 70
Pobiner, Briana, 143
Pontzer, Herman, 143
postmillennialism, 153–54, 197n8
Power, Michael, 132
powerlifting competition, 103–5
premillennialism, 153–55, 197n8
Pronger, Brian, 148–49
Protestantism, 26–27, 31, 191n33; American, 64, 65, 153, 197n8
psychology: anthropology and, 51, 191n34; cultural Christianity and American, 51; redemption and American, 51–52; secularism of American, 51; self-help, 63, 64, 65

race: apocalypse stories and, 155, 197n16, 197n18; CrossFit and, 156–63, 167; Glassman and, 156–62, 167, 168; IHME and, 158–59. *See also* Black people; white people
Reagan, Ronald, 79, 87, 109
redemption: American monomyth and, 108; American psychology on, 51–52; self and, 50, 51–52; stories, 49–50, 52
The Redemptive Self (McAdams), 50
Reeve, Christopher, 111

religion: CrossFit and, 3, 5, 23–25, 37, 113; cults and, 29–30; fitness and, 26–27; good and bad, 29–30; millennials and, 33; popular culture and, 16, 24–25; schism in history of, 150
rhabdomyolysis (rhabdo), 55, 56
Rocket Community Fitness, 157–58
Rogue, 59–60, 61, 76–78, 160
Roosevelt, Theodore, 86, 87–88
Rosman, Katherine, 160–61
Rough Riders, 88
Royce, Josiah, 34–35, 51, 188n68
Royse, Alyssa, 157–58, 166, 168
Roza, Eric, 161, 169, 172, 174, 176

salvation: American stories of, 49, 50; narratives, 50–52
salvation, Christian: American stories of redemption and, 50; confessions and testimonies of, 40–41; CrossFit salvation and, 40–41, 57; narratives, 50–52; pain and suffering in, 45–46, 49, 52; sin and, 50–51
salvation, CrossFit: Christian salvation and, 40–41, 57; in CrossFit gyms, 39–44; testimonials of, 39, 40, 41–44
Schulson, Michael, 23
science: anthropology of, 149; Aristotelian model, 130–31; audit systems and, 132; Baconian method, 131, 132; Christian imperialism and, 148; culture and, 149; deductive inquiry, 131; evolutionary, 141–46; fitness and, 133; hard, 131; inductive inquiry, 131; Western, 148, 149
science, CrossFit and, 18, 130, 139; CrossFit scientists, 196n15; evolutionary, 141–43, 145–46; fitness definitions and, 135–37, 140; Glassman and, 133–37, 142, 146–48, 149, 196n15; vigilante, 146–48, 149
secularism: American institutions and, 17; American psychology and, 51; CrossFit gyms and, 28; secular redemption stories, 52
self: American, 50, 52; redemption and, 50, 51–52; suffering self, 52, 189n10
self-help, 63–66
self-help books, 64–66
settler Christian colonialism, 50, 82, 85; afterlives of, 8, 178; CrossFit and afterlives of, 8; Indigenous people and, 86, 94; violence of, 86, 87, 93–95; wake of, 176
settler-rangers and militias, 88, 193n14
sexism, of CrossFit HQ, 160–61, 167, 168
Sharpe, Christina, 4, 176
sheroes (female heroes), 107, 110
sin and salvation narrative, 50–51
60 Minutes, "King of CrossFit" feature, 1–2, 5–8, 18, 103
slavery's wake, 176
Slotkin, Richard, 87, 89, 91, 93, 94
Smith, Christian, 17
Spencer, Herbert, 145
sport research, 15–16
Starker, Steven, 63, 64, 65
State Policy Network Conference, 14, 59, 61, 75–76
Strathern, Marilyn, 132–33, 141
Strumpf, Andy, 160, 167
suffering: self as, 52, 189n10. *See also* pain and suffering
sugar industry, 147, 149
superheroes, American, 16, 18; Christianity and, 113; comics and, 108, 109, 112; frontier heroes and, 89; monomyth of, 108, 115, 124; post-9/11 movies and, 109; white males as, 108–9, 113; whiteness of, 112–13
superheroes, CrossFit, 175; Hero WODs and, 16, 106; lifestyle, 109; post-9/11, 109; whiteness of, 7–8; women as, 111
Superman, 111
Sutton, Matthew, 153–54

T2B. *See* toes-to-bar
Taylor, Frederick, 132
television talk shows, 63
ter Kuile, Casper, 23, 33
thruster, 183
Thurston, Angie, 23, 33
Time, 23
Tocqueville, Alexis de, 16, 17
toes-to-bar (T2B), 126–27, 183
training and courses: coach training, 67; CrossFit Defense, 100; Level 1 Training Course, 10; self preservation focus of, 177
Turner, Frederick Jackson, 84–87, 89, 102, 193n6
Turtiainen, Riikka, 120
Twight, Mark, 111

Ulrich, Madeline, 24
United States (US): Christianity and foundation of, 16–17, 185n16; imperialism of, 95; militarism of, 79–80; 9/11 attacks and violence of, 95; popularity of CrossFit in, 2, 3; present day CrossFit in, 174–75; violence and, 93–95. *See also specific American topics*
US military, 2; frontier and, 82–83, 91, 96; heroes of, 89, 95–96
US military, CrossFit and: CrossFit gyms and, 91, 97–98; CrossFitters from, 97; fitness and, 63, 78–80, 90–91, 96–97, 100, 101; frontier and, 82–83, 91, 102; Glassman and, 96–97, 162; popularity, 96; post-9/11, 109, 162. *See also* Hero WODs

violence: American culture and, 93, 94; American frontier and, 82–84, 86–87, 89, 93–95, 192n1; CrossFit and, 101, 162, 163, 194n42; frontier myth and, 93–94; settler Christian colonialism and, 86, 87, 93–95; US and, 93–95; vigilante, 95; of white males, 35, 93, 94

Wagner, Rachel, 101
wake: of America, 4, 13, 16, 185n12; of settler Christian colonialism, 176; of slavery, 176. *See also* Christianity's wake
Weber, Max, 16, 17
Wellness Challenge, 43
Wertsch, James, 4, 7
white males: alienation of, 36; as American superheroes, 108–9, 113; apocalypse and elite, 151; CrossFit ethos and bravado of, 94; CrossFit gym and, 70, 80; frontier and, 83, 84, 91, 93, 193n5; imperialism of Christian, 8, 94; response to the Other of, 94; violence of, 35, 93, 94
whiteness: Americans and, 113; of American superheroes, 112–13; Christianity and, 113; of CrossFit body, 112, 113; of CrossFit superheroes, 7–8; of CrossFitters, 14, 37; heteronormative, 112, 113; Indigenous people and, 85
white people: apocalypticism of evangelical, 154–55, 197n18; Christian heteronormative, 113; CrossFit and, 113, 163, 168; CrossFit Games and, 163. *See also* race
white supremacy, 8, 112; CrossFit and, 161–62; eugenics and, 113, 145; rugged individualism and, 178; survival of fittest and, 145–46
Wild West, CrossFit and, 82, 83
Winfrey, Oprah, 63, 65–66
WOD (workout of the day), 9, 10, 184; pain and suffering in, 47, 54–55, 57; partner, 53–54, 57. *See also* Hero WODs
Wolf, Robb, 142, 144
women, frontier and, 122
women CrossFitters, 103; bodies of, 119, 121; CrossFit Games and, 116, 119, 120; as CrossFit heroes, 117–18, 122, 124; hegemonic masculinity and, 120–21; heteronormative femininity and, 119–20, 122; life changes of, 104–6, 116–17; as sheroes, 107, 110; as superheroes, 111

Wonder Woman, 111
work capacity, 133–34, 135, 136
workouts: AMRAP, 195n2; logging, 128–30
workouts, CrossFit, 1–2, 6–7, 125, 127–28; anthropological research, 8–15, 186n18; benchmark, 121–22; BTWB and, 129; curious, 9–10; as deadly, 36; *Fight Club* and, 36–37; Fran, 10, 183; functional movements in, 141; The Girls, 10, 121–22, 163, 183; injuries from, 55–56; marathon row, 150–51; masculinity and, 36–37; MetCon, 9, 183; pain and suffering in, 12, 40, 44, 46–49, 54–58; for time, 183; 21-15-9, 126, 184; violence and, 163. *See also* WOD

Young Men's Christian Associations (YMCAs), 27

Ziniewicz, Atom, 114–15
zombie apocalypse, 28, 151, 152, 155, 188n45

ABOUT THE AUTHOR

KATIE ROSE HEJTMANEK is Professor of Anthropology and of Children and Youth Studies at Brooklyn College, CUNY. She is the author of *Friendship, Love, and Hip Hop* and coeditor of *Gender and Power in Strength Sports*. She is also a world and national champion in masters Olympic weightlifting.